SOUND FIELD AMPLIFICATION

APPLICATIONS TO SPEECH PERCEPTION AND CLASSROOM ACOUSTICS

Second Edition

SOUND FIELD AMPLIFICATION
APPLICATIONS TO SPEECH PERCEPTION AND CLASSROOM ACOUSTICS
Second Edition

Carl Crandell, PhD

Department of Communication Sciences and Disorders

University of Florida

Joseph Smaldino, PhD

Department of Communicative Disorders

Northern Illinois University

Carol Flexer, PhD

School of Communicative Disorders

University of Akron

THOMSON

DELMAR LEARNING

Australia   Canada   Mexico   Singapore   Spain   United Kingdom   United States

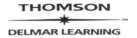

THOMSON
™
DELMAR LEARNING

Sound Field Amplification: Applications to Speech Perception and Classroom Acoustics, 2nd Edition

by Carl Crandell, PhD, Joseph Smaldino, PhD, and Carol Flexer, PhD

Vice President,
Health Care Business Unit:
William Brottmiller

Editorial Director:
Cathy L. Esperti

Acquisitions Editor:
Kalen Conerly

Developmental Editor:
Laurie Traver

Marketing Director:
Jennifer McAvey

Marketing Coordinator:
Chris Manion

Editorial Assistants:
James Duncan
Elizabeth Howe

Project Editor:
David Buddle

Production Coordinator:
Jessica McNavich

Art and Design Coordinator:
Christi DiNinni

Art and Design Specialist:
Robert Plante

COPYRIGHT © 2005, 1995 by Thomson Delmar Learning, a part of The Thomson Corporation. Thomson, the star logo, and Delmar Learning are trademarks used herein under license.

Printed in Canada
1 2 3 4 5 6 7 XXX 08 07 06 05 04

For more information, contact Thomson Delmar Learning,
5 Maxwell Drive,
Clifton Park, NY 12065-2919
Or you can visit our Internet site at
http://www.delmarlearning.com

Library of Congress cataloguing-in-publication data

Crandell, Carl C.
 Sound field amplification : applications to speech perception and classroom acoustics / Carl Crandell, Joseph Smaldino, Carol Flexer.—2nd ed.
   p.   cm.
Rev. ed. of: Sound field FM amplification, 1995.
 Includes bibliographical references and index.
ISBN 1-4018-5145-2
 1. School buildings—Acoustics—United States. 2. Auditory perception in children. 3. Classroom management—United States. I. Smaldino, Joseph J. II. Flexer, Carol Ann. III. Crandell, Carl C. Sound field FM amplification. IV. Title.
LB3241.5.C73 2004
371.6'2—dc22
                        2004050163

NOTICE TO THE READER

To the students, born and unborn, who by oversight or neglect suffer the consequences of inappropriate classroom acoustics.

CONTENTS

FOREWORD

I was delighted when I was asked to write the foreword to the first edition of this book. It covered a topic that cried out for a scholarly publication, one that would not only cover the facts but also convey the crucial importance of this technology for children in our schools. I am just as delighted now to write the foreword to this edition. However, as I look over what I wrote for the first edition, I find that there is little that I would want to change or withdraw (well, maybe a few typographical and grammatical errors!). Given what I discussed in the earlier edition, then, what can I possibly add that is new now?

Conceptually, there is actually nothing to add. Quite clearly, children still have to hear in classrooms in order to learn. That has not changed, and it will not. Most classrooms still do not present acoustically friendly learning environments. We knew then and we know now that sound field amplification systems can help convert a stressful situation into one more acceptable for learning. If we want to increase the likelihood that children will learn the material being presented by teachers, then we must make certain they hear what the teacher says. The more that they hear, the more they are likely to learn. This is not to say that developments in the area have remained stagnant. Since the days the first edition appeared, a great deal of additional information can be brought to bear to support the concept even more.

There is now a clearer understanding of the impact of poor classroom acoustics on the performance of children—all kinds of children, including those with normal hearing and those exhibiting a multitude of conditions—than what we had ten years ago when the first edition was written. This clearer understanding has resulted in new national standards regarding acceptable acoustical conditions in classrooms. These are reviewed and discussed in the book. This is a major step forward. And, I would like to note, it is a step that probably would not have taken place without the intense, and sometimes even annoying, efforts of some parents who have tried to ensure a reasonable learning environment for their children. It was they, I believe, who moved the issue onto the national agenda. The power of parents once again has been displayed!

Ten years ago, ensuring the proper dispersal of the amplified signal within the classroom was a bit chancy. Now we are able to improve our goal of ensuring a positive speech-to-noise ratio at all locations within a classroom. Before, as the title of the first edition indicated, only FM technology could be used to provide an amplified version of the teacher's voice. Sometimes, in some places, this could not easily be achieved because of RF interference, either originating from the outside or from other RF systems within the building. Now we have infrared sound field systems that are less susceptible to this type of interference. This has opened the door for the possibility of a sound field system in *every* classroom in which it is needed.

Ten years ago, it was the rare classroom that could boast a sound field system. Now it is a recognized educational tool appearing in more and more classrooms around the country, but still not enough. Judging from the results of the studies supporting the concept, many more classrooms in our country could benefit from the inclusion of sound field technology. So why isn't it more widely used? Why is there still so much resistance to employing this valuable tool in more settings?

Money is certainly one reason. Still, as several projects have demonstrated, the use of sound field technology in classrooms can actually save money by reducing the number of students who require a special education component. But this is not the major reason. The major reason for resistance to its use lies in the fact that decision makers in schools judge the appropriateness of the acoustical environment from the evidence of their own ears rather than from the children in the classroom. It is very difficult for people with perfectly normal hearing to critically analyze the acoustical conditions existing in a classroom when they themselves have no difficulty hearing in that same environment. I have personally had this experience numerous times over the years: trying to carry on a conversation with a teacher in a noisy classroom and finding it difficult, and sometimes impossible, to do so given my hearing loss. Yet, the teacher could follow my conversation with relative ease.

Still, short of requiring a hearing loss of every teacher, there has to be a way of conveying the crucial necessity of a good speech-to-noise ratio in classrooms. This book is one powerful way to do this. The rationale, the evidence, and the technical details are all here. Any reasonable person who reads this material will be convinced. Also, we know that it is not only the hearing-impaired child who can benefit, but any child who has a shaky command of the language or who is unable to withstand the impact of even relatively minor noise and reverberent conditions.

Above all, we must acknowledge that it is through the sense of hearing that most children can best learn language. It is through the auditory channel that they internalize the phonological categories that they then apply to the reading process. The implications are obvious: why not provide children with the clearest, most distortion-free sample of their teacher's speech? They will hear better, behave better, and be better educated. The trouble is, it seems too simple, too good to be true. We have somehow been conditioned to believe that a solution has to be complex in order to be effective. But sometimes, it is the obvious solution that has the most validity.

What readers of this book should understand is that the contributors are not simply dry academic types, writing their prose in an acceptable "scholarly" fashion. These people, all of whom I know, are more than first-rate professionals; they are dedicated clinicians who have personally seen what can be done with the effective use of sound field amplification. They have personally seen (and often investigated) the improvements in speech perception wrought by an improved speech-to-noise ratio. They have seen academic performance increase and behavior improve. And they have listened to teacher after teacher laud this technology, and not just for children, but for themselves as well. They no longer finish the school day with a hoarse voice!

For the contributors, therefore, the topic is more than just an academic exercise, although the science and facts are here and are irrefutable. For them, it is a mission to which they have devoted much of their lives. Their passion may not always be evident in their academic prose, but it is there. They believe, as I do, that this technology is one of the most powerful educational tools we have available for the children in our schools.

I would not go so far as to say that a sound field system belongs in every classroom, but I will say that every classroom should at least be evaluated to determine whether one is needed. The evaluation itself would be a sign of respect for the role that the sense of hearing plays in our lives. This is the overarching theme that is the central focus of this book and is implicit in every chapter.

Mark Ross, PhD
Professor Emeritus
University of Connecticut

PREFACE

PURPOSE

The purpose of this second edition has expanded in an exciting way from the first edition. We still intend the book to be a comprehensive and cohesive textbook and handbook for the use of small FM and infrared sound field systems; however, we are extending the focus to include critical information about speech perception and classroom acoustics. In addition, the theoretical and practical areas have been enriched. In order to provide a broader focus on application of this information to real situations and scenarios, we have included more examples in this edition. Besides the popular worksheets and checklists present in the first edition, we have added "Key Points" and "Discussion Topics" to each chapter. We especially hope that the discussion topics will broaden and deepen knowledge about the content of each chapter and be a guide for students.

AUDIENCE

This book continues to be written for the large number of students, professionals, and consumers who might use and benefit from sound field amplification systems and for those who desire information about speech perception and classroom acoustics. Readers encompass students (audiology—AuD, speech-language pathology, special education, and general education students), audiologists, speech-language pathologists, school administrators, classroom teachers, special education teachers, teachers of children who are deaf or hard of hearing, parent-teacher associations, parents, civic groups, and equipment manufacturers.

BOOK CONTENT

In this edition, we have again tried to separate the theoretical from the practical issues surrounding sound field amplification. The reason for this is that students and professionals who intend to learn about and obtain sound field systems for their schools first need to show the need for this technology. There is a research basis predicated on speech perception for amplifying general education classrooms as well as special education classrooms. Next, interested persons need to know how to select, install, use, and maintain this equipment as well as how to manage classroom acoustics and pupils' listening skills. This book has been designed to address all of these issues.

Section A

Section A of this book details the theoretical foundation that supports the use of sound field systems in classrooms. A thorough understanding of that foundation is necessary for the appropriate utilization of sound field technology. Therefore, this book begins by building the theoretical scaffolding that bridges to practical applications. Chapter 1 focuses on the rationale for the use of sound field systems in classrooms. Although in the theoretical section, much of the information provided is useful and practical when trying to educate stakeholders about the need for classroom amplification. In Chapter 2 we welcome a new contributor, Arthur Boothroyd, who presents a very thorough discussion of how room acoustics affect speech perception. Graphics and examples are used extensively to elucidate this complex topic. Chapter 3 reprises and expands the popular speech-perception model from the first edition, which provides an acoustic context for speech and language development. Chapter 4 presents an overview of the populations of children who have more difficulty learning in a classroom environment than do typical children. The theoretical section is concluded with Chapter 5 in which a comprehensive literature review provides a research direction for the interested student, professional, and consumer.

Section B

Section B takes the theoretical foundation that was developed in the first part of this book and transfers it to practical situations. Sound field technology is only as good as its application. Chapter 6 overviews new acoustic standards and discusses classroom acoustic measurement techniques. Chapter 7 focuses on the acoustical modifications that can be made in classrooms so that they will more closely conform to desirable acoustic conditions. Chapter 8 addresses the nitty-gritty of installing a sound field amplification system in a classroom. Chapter 9 follows with considerations and suggestions for enhancing listening skills and addresses how listening strategies can enable teachers and pupils to make maximum use of sound field technology. Chapter 10 brings to light the importance of measuring efficacy after a sound field system is installed and presents some instruments that might be used for that purpose. Chapter 11 provides numerous suggestions for marketing and obtaining funding for sound field systems. Chapter 12 overviews the laws and regulations that govern the utilization of sound field technology in both general education and special education classrooms and provides a rationale for policy makers.

NEW TO THIS EDITION

Because we intend this book to be applicable as both a textbook and a hand-book, this second edition has added "Key Points" and "Discussion Topics" to each chapter. The key points help to highlight the main ideas of each chapter, and the discussion topics promote critical thinking. In addition, information has been updated and the focus has been extended to include critical data about speech perception and classroom acoustics. New sound field technologies and acoustic standards are included in these updates. Additional appendices include sample efficacy forms. Finally, in order to provide a broader focus on application of information to real situations, case studies have been included in this edition.

Sound field technology, FM and infrared, plays an increasingly important role in the education of our children. In this day and age of "No Child Left Behind," understanding speech-perception processes and acoustic accessibility is critical. This book can serve as a textbook and guide to creating and managing the acoustic environment and listening capabilities of all students.

REVIEWERS

We would like to thank the following educators and professionals for their thoughtful comments, feedback, and insight as they reviewed our manuscript:

Carole E. Johnson, PhD
Department of Communication Disorders
Auburn University
Auburn, Alabama

Carol Mackersie, PhD
School of Speech, Language and Hearing Sciences
San Diego State University
San Diego, California

Susan Prendergast, PhD
Department of Speech Pathology and Audiology
Illinois State University
Normal, Illinois

Claudia Updike, PhD
Department of Speech Pathology and Audiology
Ball State University
Muncie, Indiana

CONTRIBUTORS

Laurie A. Allen, MA
Educational Audiologist
Keystone Area Education Agency
Dubuque, Iowa

Karen L. Anderson, PhD
Audiology Consultant
Florida Department of Health,
    Children's Medical Services
Bureau of Early Interventions
Tallahassee, Florida

Arthur Boothroyd, PhD
Distinguished Professor Emeritus
City University of New York
New York, New York

Carolyn Edwards, MClSc, MBA
Director, Auditory Management
    Services
Toronto, Ontario, Canada

Brian M. Kreisman, PhD
Department of Communication
    Sciences and Disorders
Institute for the Advanced Study of
    Communication Processes
University of Florida
Gainesville, Florida

Nicole V. Kreisman, MA
Department of Communication
    Sciences and Disorders
Institute for the Advanced Study of
    Communication Processes
University of Florida
Gainesville, Florida

Gail Gegg Rosenberg, MS
1450, Inc.
Sarasota, Florida

AUTHORS

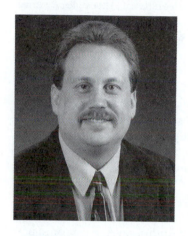

Carl C. Crandell received his bachelor's degree and master's degree from Florida State University and obtained his PhD with honors from Vanderbilt University in 1989. He taught audiology and hearing sciences at the Callier Center for Communication Disorders at the University of Texas at Dallas for five years and currently is Professor of Audiology at the University of Florida. Dr. Crandell's research has focused on the areas of listening, communication, and speech perception in pediatric, hearing-impaired, and elderly listeners. He has also conducted considerable research on hearing aids and classroom amplification technologies. This research has led to numerous publications, presentations at scientific meetings, book chapters, and grant funding.

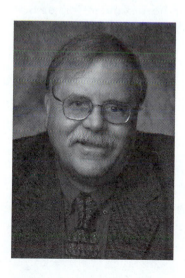

Joseph J. Smaldino received his bachelor's degree in biological sciences from Union College, his MS degree in hearing science from the University of Connecticut, and his PhD in Audiology from the University of Florida. He has been the director of a Veterans Administration Audiology clinic, a department head, and is a professor of Audiology. He has more than twenty-five years of clinical experience. He has been the national president of the Academy of Rehabilitative Audiology and the Educational Audiology Association. Dr. Smaldino is a Fellow of the American Speech-Language-Hearing Association, has received the 2001–2002 University of Northern Iowa Distinguished Scholar Award, and has been a

Fulbright research fellow. For more than twenty years, he has researched the effects of hearing loss on speech perception and has studied the effects of various electroacoustic parameters of hearing aids on improving perception. Recent research interest has focused on the effects of classroom acoustics on speech perception.

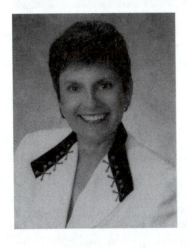

Carol Flexer received a PhD in Audiology from Kent State University in 1982. She has been at the University of Akron for twenty-three years where she is a professor of Audiology in the School of Speech-Language Pathology and Audiology and the Northeast Ohio Au.D. Consortium (NOAC). Special areas of expertise include pediatric and educational audiology. She has lectured internationally, authored more than one hundred publications, including a book titled *Facilitating Hearing and Listening in Young Children* (first and second editions), and co-edited two books: *How the Student with Hearing Loss Can Succeed in College* (first and second editions) and *Sound-Field FM Amplification: Theory and Practical Applications* (first edition). She is a past president of the Educational Audiology Association, a past board member of Auditory-Verbal International, Inc. (Cert. AVT), and a past president of the American Academy of Audiology. For her research and advocacy for children with hearing loss, Dr. Flexer was a recipient of the Volta Award, the most prestigious award conferred by the Alexander Graham Bell Association for the Deaf and Hard of Hearing.

ACKNOWLEGMENTS

Carl Crandell: I would like to thank the good Lord for giving me such wonderful colleagues as Carol and Joe to work with. You both are a real blessing! I would also like to thank my beautiful wife, Lorraine, and daughter, Danielle, for always being there for me. Finally, I would like to thank Andrew, Nicole, and Brian for reading and editing what seemed like several thousand drafts of this book. Thanks, guys!

Joseph Smaldino: I would like to thank all of the professionals and mentors who came before, published their results and ideas, and exalted us to follow in their footsteps and exceed expectations. Carl and Carol, you are magical people and I am honored to call each of you coauthor, colleague, and friend. For Sharon, whose quiet comfort and love has and will always be an inspiration. Finally, for my sons, Matt and Ben, who are serving in the military during these troubled times.

Carol Flexer: I would like to express gratitude and appreciation to Carl Crandell and Joe Smaldino. They really are the dream team. I treasure their lifelong friendship and dedication. A special acknowledgment needs to be extended to Mark Ross. He has been and continues to be an inspiration to me. And finally, I would like to thank my dear husband, Pete, my amazing children Heather, Hillari, and David, and my six precious grandchildren for their consistent enthusiasm and love of life.

From Carol and Joseph to Carl: Yet again, you did good.

THEORETICAL APPLICATIONS OF SOUND FIELD AMPLIFICATION

CHAPTER 1

Rationale for the Use of Sound Field Systems in Classrooms: The Basis of Teacher In-Services

Carol Flexer, PhD

KEY POINTS

- Hearing is a primary way that information is entered into a student's brain in a classroom; data input precedes data processing.
- Key educational issues that typically have been ignored are the listening demands placed on children in poor acoustic environments, compounded by the immature listening skills that children bring to a classroom situation.
- Hearing is a first-order event in a mainstream classroom; if a child cannot clearly hear spoken instruction, the entire premise of the educational system is undermined.
- Sound distribution systems must be featured when discussing the classroom listening environment because these systems improve the sound-to-noise ratio.
- Without basic detection of intelligible speech, comprehension of complex concepts is impossible; sound field systems enhance detection.

Sometimes the simplest concepts are the most profound, and the simplest solutions are the most powerful. One simple concept is that in typical classrooms, children need to hear in order to learn. And, as Dr. Mark Ross explains in the foreword, the better children hear, the more they likely will learn. One

3

simple solution is to amplify and evenly distribute the teacher's speech throughout the classroom so that all children can better hear spoken instruction. This book is about understanding the critical nature of classroom listening, literacy, and learning, and about managing and enhancing the educational environment.

One of the most challenging learning domains is the classroom. Children spend much of their time in noisy classroom environments where teachers demand constant, detailed listening to critical instruction that is spoken far from students.

There are two major factors that affect auditory learning in the classroom: the hearing of the child and the classroom environment. Additional variables include the speech of the teacher and pupils, and their relative positions in the room. However, the speech of talkers is filtered through the physical environment of the room and the auditory system of the listener; therefore, these two variables are of primary consideration.

The purpose of this chapter is to provide a rationale for the use of sound field technology by discussing how the hearing of the child and the classroom acoustic environment impact listening, literacy, and learning. In addition, a guide for teacher in-services will be offered.

THE WORLD HAS CHANGED

There is a big-picture perspective to be considered when discussing classroom learning. Because the United States now has an information/knowledge-based economy, a sizeable proportion of our workforce needs to have high levels of spoken language and literacy skills in order to keep our country viable and progressing (Alter, 1999).

The world has changed rapidly during the past ten years, and the pace of change is escalating (Johnson, 1998). Technology is the driving force for change, and workforce skills need to keep pace with the change. The children who are in today's classrooms will be the leaders, contributors, and voters of the years 2030, 2040, and 2050. We are creating that future by instilling in our children a solid foundation of transferable skills and a lifelong love for learning. In this era of rapid change, proficient literacy skills will be necessary for our children to be able to manage the constant updating of their knowledge base (Robertson, 2002; Trelease, 2001).

Literacy

Reading has a strong auditory foundation (Chermak & Musiek, 1997; Robertson, 2000). Specifically, phonological awareness, the knowledge that language is composed of a system of words and syllables, is one of the primary building blocks for developing literacy skills. Phonemic awareness is the knowledge that words themselves are composed of individual sounds called phonemes. Clearly, phonemic awareness is an auditory skill dealing with the sounds of spoken language. Therefore, the better that speech sounds can be heard, the stronger will be the foundation for literacy (Robertson, 2000).

Because of the need for our children to keep pace with the changing world, literacy is a national priority (Trelease, 2001). We face substantial challenges. In the year 2000, data showed that the percentage of fourth-grade students reading at or above proficient, the level identified by the National Assessment Governing Board (NAGB) as the goal for all students, increased only slightly to 32% from 29% in 1992 (National Center for Education Statistics, 2001). These data mean that only about a third of fourth graders in the United States can read at their grade level. Moreover, while scores for the nation's highest performing students have improved over the years, scores of the lowest performing students have declined.

Of critical importance is the fact that there has been no closing of the education gap between students who are white and students who are minorities. Specifically, in the year 2000, 40% of fourth-grade white students and 46% of Asian/Pacific Islander students could read at or above the proficient achievement level. However, only 12% African-American students, 16% of Hispanic students, and 17% of Native American students could read at or above the proficient achievement level (National Center for Education Statistics, 2001). According to these data, large numbers of children who are minorities do not possess the literacy skills that would enable them to have flexibility and dynamism in the workforce.

Clearly, we are not educating whole segments of our school population, and we have not been for the last ten years. Consequently, the gap between rich and poor is now greater than at any time since the Great Depression (Alter, 1999). The richest 2.7 million Americans now have as much money as the poorest 100 million, and these trends are being fueled by technology and the notion that what you earn depends on what you learn.

So, what is missing in our classrooms? What have we failed to consider? The neglected concepts as proposed in this chapter include the immature listening abilities of children and the poor listening environments in classrooms.

THE CHILD: HEARING AND LISTENING

We "hear" with the brain. The ears are just a way in. The problem with hearing loss and with poor auditory environments is that intact sound is barred from reaching the brain. The purpose of having favorable listening environments and amplification technologies is to channel complete words efficiently and effectively to the brain.

Recent studies in brain development show that stimulation of the auditory centers of the brain is critical (Berlin & Weyand, 2003; Boothroyd, 1997; Chermak & Musiek, 1997; Sharma, Dorman, & Spahr, 2002; Sloutsky & Napolitano, 2003). Sensory stimulation influences the actual growth and organization of auditory brain pathways (Bhatnagar, 2002; Sharma, Dorman, & Spahr, 2002; Sloutsky & Napolitano, 2003). Therefore, anything that can be done to access, grow, and program those important and powerful auditory centers of the brain with acoustic detail expands children's opportunities for enhancement of life function. A child's hearing loss, no matter how minimal, can be a roadblock to getting sufficient sounds to the brain unless amplification technologies are used. Amplification is really about brain stimulation with subsequent brain growth.

It is important to recognize that children are not small adults. They are not able to listen like adults listen. Indeed, children bring a different listening to a communicative and learning situation than do adults in two main ways. First, human auditory brain structure is not fully mature until about age fifteen; thus, a child does not bring a complete neurological system to a listening situation (Bhatnagar, 2002; Boothroyd, 1997; Chermak & Musiek, 1997). Second, children do not have the years of language and life experience that enable adults to fill in the gaps of missed or inferred information (such filling in of gaps is called auditory/cognitive closure). Therefore, because children require more complete, detailed auditory information than adults, in whom sounds enters a developed brain, all children need a quieter room and a louder signal (Anderson, 2001). The goal is to develop the brains of children.

Large populations of children who often are not identified are those with hearing problems caused by middle ear dysfunction. Indeed, the incidence of children with persistent minimal to mild hearing impairments caused by otitis media may be much higher than school screenings lead us to believe. Hearing screening environments in schools typically have less than ideal levels of ambient noise, causing hearing to be screened at 20 to 35 dB hearing level (HL). When 15 dB HL is used as the criterion for identifying an educationally significant hearing impairment, the numbers of identified kindergarten and first-grade children increase dramatically. A study conducted in Putnam County, Ohio, found that 43% of primary-level students failed a 15 dB HL hearing screen on any given day, and about 75% of primary-level children in classes for children with learning disabilities failed a 15 dB hearing screening (Flexer, 1989). Another study projected that 14.9% of U.S. school children—that's about 8 million school children!—have hearing loss that can impact their educational progress (Niskar et al., 1998).

Typical mainstream classrooms are auditory-verbal environments; instruction is presented through the teacher's spoken communication (Berg, 1993). The underlying assumption is that children can hear clearly and attend to the teacher's speech. Thus, children in a mainstream classroom, whether or not they have hearing problems, must be able to hear the teacher in order for learning to occur. If children cannot consistently and clearly hear the teacher, the major premise of the educational system is undermined.

Levels of Auditory Skill Development

There is a great deal involved in "hearing" the teacher. Erber (1982) was one of the first to identify the levels of auditory skill development associated with "hearing and listening," and Ling (2002) has expanded on them.

- Detection: This is the lowest, least sophisticated level of auditory skill development. Detection refers to the presence and absence of sound. Obtaining pure tone thresholds is a detection task.
- Discrimination: This involves distinguishing between two speech sounds. An example of a discrimination task would be noting if *da* and *tha* are the same or different.
- Recognition: This is a closed-set task that involves selecting a target from a known list of alternatives.
- Identification: This is an open-set task that involves noting a target from an infinite set of alternatives.
- Comprehension: This is the highest level of auditory skill development. Comprehension is achieved when one can answer questions, follow directions, and hold conversations.

It is critical to note that without basic detection, none of the higher levels of auditory processing are available. Therefore, comprehension, the goal of classroom instruction, is completely dependent on the initial detection of individual phonemes that comprise the spoken message. Challenging acoustic environments, hearing problems, and the immature listening skills of children all compromise detection. Without detection, there can be no comprehension. Without comprehension, literacy will be sabotaged.

Word-Sound Distinctions

Elliott, Hammer, and Scholl conducted a key study in 1989. They evaluated primary-level children with normal hearing and found that the ability to perform fine-grained auditory discrimination tasks (e.g., to hear *pa* and *ba* as different syllables) correctly classified 80% of the children in their study either as progressing normally or as having language-learning difficulties. The conclusion is that auditory discrimination is associated with the development of basic academic competencies that are critical for success in school. Auditory discrimination cannot occur unless basic detection is first available. The young child who cannot hear (detect) phonemic distinctions is at risk for academic failure.

Audibility versus Intelligibility

The ability to detect the presence of speech but not identify individual components is called audibility. The lower frequencies, 250 Hz and 500 Hz, carry audibility. These frequencies contain about 90% of the energy of speech but only approximately 10% of the intelligibility. These are the power sounds. On the other hand, the ability to discriminate individual phonemes, to hear word-sound distinctions, is defined as intelligibility. Intelligibility is carried by high-frequency consonant sounds. The frequencies 2,000 Hz and 4,000 Hz contain approximately 90% of the intelligibility of speech but only about 10% of the energy of speech (Bess & Humes, 2003). They are weak sounds that are easily masked by a noisy environment or dissipated by distance. If a child lacks persistent intelligibility (is unable to discriminate *walked* from *walks,* for example) because of poor attending skills, an auditory processing problem, poor classroom acoustics, or a hearing impairment of any degree, he or she will not learn appropriate semantic distinctions unless deliberate intervention occurs.

Invisible Acoustic Filter Effect of Hearing Problems

The primacy of hearing in the communicative and educational process tends to be underestimated because hearing loss itself is invisible. The effects of hearing loss often are associated with problems or causes other than hearing impairment (Flexer, 1999; Ross, Brackett, & Maxon, 1991). For example, when a child is off-task or cannot keep up with the rapid pace of class discussion, the cause of that child's behavior may be attributed to noncompliant behavior, attention problems, or slow learning rather than to hearing problems.

One cannot "see" a hearing problem; therefore, it is easy to confuse the causal hearing loss with the negative consequences of the hearing impairment. Hearing problems act like an invisible acoustic filter that interferes with incoming sound (Ling, 2002). In addition to a reduction in loudness, sounds are often smeared together or filtered out entirely. Speech, therefore, might be audible but not intelligible. A child with a hearing problem might be able to hear the presence of speech (audibility) but not be able to hear clearly enough to identify one speech sound as distinct from another. Words such as "invitation" and "vacation" might sound the same. It is not difficult to imagine what such word confusions could do to a child's vocabulary and conceptual language development.

This acoustic filter effect is the beginning and the cause of an entire chain of negative events. If speech sounds are not heard clearly, then one cannot speak clearly (one speaks what one hears) unless deliberate intervention occurs. The second step in the chain involves reading ability. If one does not have good spoken language skills, then reading, which is a secondary linguistic function, also will suffer (Robertson, 2000). Said another way, we speak because we hear, and we read because we speak. If reading skills are below average, an individual will have difficulty performing academically. Limited literacy leads to a reduction in professional options and subsequent opportunities for independent function as an adult. The cause of this entire unfortunate chain of events is the ambiguous, invisible, underestimated, and often untreated acoustic filter effect of hearing problems. Until the primary issue of poor classroom listening environments and the unsophisticated listening skills of children are understood and managed, thus providing the brain with access to detailed sound, intervention at the secondary levels of spoken language, reading, and academics likely will be ineffective.

Computer Analogy

One way to explain the negative effects of poor classroom acoustics on literacy and academic performance is to use a computer analogy (Flexer, 1999). Data input precedes data output. A child must have information or data in order to learn. Information is entered into the brain through the auditory system. If data are entered inaccurately, as with having one's fingers on the wrong keys of a computer keyboard or having a broken keyboard, then the child will have inaccurate, incomplete, and unreliable data to process. Is it reasonable to expect a child to learn sophisticated spoken communication and to develop literacy skills when the information that reaches the brain is deficient?

Favorable classroom acoustics and sound field amplification are analogous to having a better keyboard. The goal of having an acoustically accessible classroom is to provide the best, most consistent and reliable keyboard for instructional data entry. The better a child can detect word-sound distinctions, the better opportunity a child will have for the development of academic competencies.

Once hearing problems are identified and barriers to the clear reception of classroom instruction are removed, analogous to the provision of the best possible keyboard, what happens to all of the previously entered inaccurate and deficient information? Do inaccurate data convert automatically to correct information? Unfortunately, missing data need to be reentered and inaccurate data need to be corrected.

Managing the classroom listening environment, beginning with detection, is the crucial first step in the learning chain; providing an accurate and reliable keyboard is the prerequisite step to clear data entry. Once auditory brain centers have been accessed, a child has an opportunity to learn spoken language as the basis for developing literacy and academic skills and acquiring knowledge about the world.

Passive Learning, Overhearing, and Distance Hearing

Inappropriate classroom acoustics can interfere with distance hearing. Distance hearing is the distance over which speech sounds are intelligible and not merely audible. Noisy environments and/or hearing problems of any type and degree reduce the distance over which speech sounds are intelligible (Boothroyd, 2002). Typically, the greater the hearing loss, the greater the reduction in distance hearing. Reduction in distance hearing has negative consequences for classroom and life performance because distance hearing is necessary for passive learning (Flexer, 1999).

A child with a hearing problem, even a minimal one, cannot casually overhear what people are saying. Most children with normal hearing seem to absorb information from their environments if their environments are quiet; they tend to learn easily information that was not directed to them. Children with hearing problems, however, because of their reduction in distance hearing, need to be taught directly many skills and concepts that other children learn incidentally.

Additional implications of the reduction of distance hearing include lack of redundancy of instructional information and lack of access to social cues. Listening is an active, not a passive, process for children with hearing problems. Thus, active attention must be directed to appropriate sources at all times.

A child's attention will wander often during the school day, causing him or her to miss some of what is being said. Missed information can be offset partially by the use of a remote microphone in a sound field system. The remote microphone can be placed close to the speech or sound source, thereby making information available and alleviating some of the strain and effort of constant disciplined attention.

Level of Effort

Children with hearing problems, even minimal ones, typically expend a high level of effort as they attempt to learn from classroom instruction.

As Mark Ross has often stated, the problem with hearing loss is that you do not hear so well. Consequently, you hear what you think you hear, and you do not hear what you do not hear—and one does not have a perspective about missed information (Ross, Brackett, & Maxon, 1991).

THE LISTENING ENVIRONMENT OF THE CLASSROOM

Another important factor is the listening environment of the classroom. Several factors in this area are discussed below.

Speech-to-Noise Ratio

Unfortunately, children are expected to hear meaningful word-sound distinctions in unfavorable acoustic environments. They must listen to a speaker who is not close and who is moving about the room. Signal-to-noise (S/N) ratio is the relationship between a primary signal, such as the teacher's speech, and background noise. Noise is everything that conflicts with the auditory signal of choice, such as other talkers, heating or cooling systems, classroom or hall noise, playground sounds, computer noise, or wind. The quieter the room and the more favorable the S/N ratio, the clearer the auditory signal will be for the brain. The farther the listener is from the desired sound source and the noisier the environment, the poorer the S/N ratio and the more garbled the signal will be for the brain. As stated previously, all children—especially those with hearing loss—need a quieter environment and a louder signal than adults do in order to learn (Anderson, 2001).

Adults with normal hearing and intact listening skills require a consistent S/N ratio of approximately +6 dB for the reception of intelligible speech (Bess & Humes, 2003). Children need a much more favorable S/N ratio because of their neurological immaturity and lack of life and language experience that reduces their ability to perform auditory/cognitive closure. In addition, because of internal auditory distortion, persons with any type or degree of hearing problem require a more favorable S/N ratio—about +20 dB. Due to noise, reverberation, and variations in teacher position, the S/N ratio in a typical classroom is unstable and averages out to only about +4 dB and may be 0 dB, often less than ideal even for adults with normal hearing (Crandell & Smaldino, 2002).

Rapid Speech Transmission Index

The negative effects of a typical classroom environment on the integrity of a speech signal probably have been underestimated. Leavitt and Flexer conducted a key study in 1991 to investigate this issue. They used the Bruel and Kjaer Rapid Speech Transmission Index (RASTI) to measure the effects of a classroom environment on a speechlike signal. The RASTI signal, an amplitude-modulated broadband noise centered at 500 and 2,000 Hz, was transmitted from the RASTI transmitter to the RASTI receiver that was placed at seventeen different locations around a typical occupied classroom. The RASTI score is a measure of the integrity of signals as they are propagated across the physical space. A perfect reproduction of the RASTI signal at the receiver has a score of 1.0.

Results showed that sound degradation occurred as the RASTI receiver was moved away from the RASTI transmitter as reflected by a decrease in

RASTI scores (Leavitt & Flexer, 1991). In the front-row center seat, the most preferred seat, the RASTI score dropped to 0.83. In the back row, the RASTI score was only 0.55, reflecting a loss of 45% of equivalent speech intelligibility in a quiet, occupied classroom. Only at the six-inch reference position could a perfect RASTI score of 1.0 be obtained. Note that the RASTI score represents only the loss of speech fidelity that might be expected at the student's ear or hearing aid microphone port in a quiet classroom. The RASTI score does not measure the additional negative effects of a child's hearing loss, weak auditory or language base, or attention problems.

Even in a front-row center seat, the loss of critical speech information is noteworthy for a child who needs accurate data entry to learn. The most sophisticated of hearing aids or cochlear implants cannot recreate those components of the speech signal that have been lost in transmission across the physical space of the classroom.

SOUND FIELD SYSTEMS—FM OR INFRARED

Sound field technology is an exciting educational tool that allows control of the acoustic environment in a classroom, thereby facilitating acoustic accessibility of teacher instruction for all children in the room (Flexer, 1998). A sound field system looks like a wireless public address system, but it is designed specifically to ensure that the entire speech signal, including the weak high-frequency consonants, reaches every child in the room. By using this technology, an entire classroom can be amplified through the use of one, two, three, or four wall- or ceiling-mounted loudspeakers.

One example of a sound field system is shown in Figure 1-1b, which is one type of FM unit that has a single, portable, column loudspeaker with a teacher microphone and a pass-around microphone for the students. Figure 1-2 in this chapter shows a student using one of these pass-around microphones.

The teacher wears a wireless microphone transmitter, just like the one worn for a personal FM unit, and her voice is sent via radio waves (FM) or light waves (infrared) to an amplifier that is connected to the loudspeakers. There are no wires connecting the teacher with the equipment. The radio or light wave link allows the teacher to move about freely, unrestricted by wires.

Proposed New Term: Sound Field Distribution System

The term "sound field distribution system" has been proposed as being more descriptive of sound field function. Some teachers, parents, and acoustical engineers interpret the labels "sound field amplification" or "classroom amplification" to mean that all sounds in the classroom are made louder. This misunderstanding may give the impression that sound is blasted into a room,

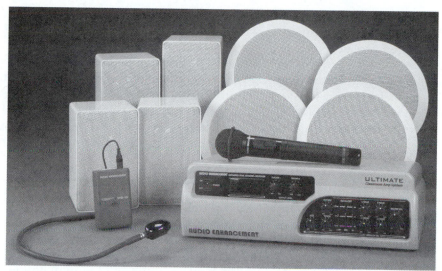

a

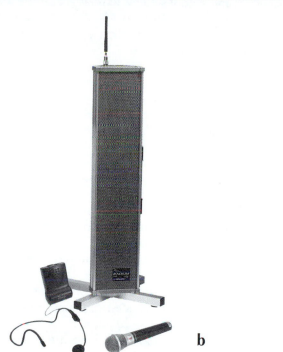

b

Figures 1-1a and 1-1b: For sound field technology, the teacher wears a wireless microphone transmitter, and her speech is sent via light waves—infrared (1a) or radio waves, FM (1b)—to an amplifier and loudspeakers. (Figure 1-1a courtesy of Audio Enhancement; Figure 1-1b courtesy of Phonic Ear, Inc.)

causing rising noise levels, interfering with instruction in adjacent rooms, and provoking anxiety in pupils. In actuality, when the equipment is installed and used appropriately, the reverse is true. The teacher's amplified voice can sound soothing as it is evenly distributed throughout the room easily, reaching every child. The room quiets as students attend to spoken instruction. In fact, the listener is aware of the sound distribution and ease of listening only when the equipment is turned off. The overall purpose of the equipment is to improve detection by having the details of spoken instruction continually reach the brains of all pupils.

Children Who Might Benefit from Sound Field Distribution Systems

It could be argued that virtually all children could benefit from sound field distribution systems because the improved S/N ratio creates a more favorable learning environment. If children could hear better, clearer, and more consistently, they would have an opportunity to learn more efficiently (Rosenberg et al., 1999). Some school systems have as a goal the amplification of every classroom in their districts (Knittel, Myott, & McClain, 2002).

No one disputes the necessity of creating a favorable visual field in a classroom. A school building never would be constructed without lights in every classroom. However, because hearing is invisible and ambiguous, the necessity of creating a favorable auditory field may be questioned by school personnel. Nevertheless, studies continue to show that sound distribution systems facilitate opportunities for improved academic performance. (See Chapter 5 of this book for a detailed listing of studies that support the use of sound distribution technology.)

The populations that seem to be especially in need of S/N ratio-enhancing technology include children with fluctuating conductive hearing impairments, unilateral hearing impairments, minimal permanent hearing impairments, auditory processing problems, cochlear implants, cognitive disorders, learning disabilities, attention problems, articulation disorders, and behavior problems.

Teachers who use sound field technology report that they also benefit. Many state that they need to use less energy projecting their voices; they have less vocal abuse and are less tired by the end of the school day. Teachers also report that the unit increases their efficiency as teachers, requiring fewer repetitions and thus allowing for more actual teaching time.

With more and more schools incorporating principles of inclusion where children who would have been in self-contained placements are in the mainstream classroom, sound field distribution systems offer a way of enhancing the classroom learning environment for the benefit of all children. It is a win-win situation.

The Issue of Literacy and Sound Field Distribution Systems

There is evidence that sound field distribution systems can improve literacy development. Numerous studies have been reported (see Chapter 5 of this book). An article by Darai (2000) found that sound field systems, when appropriately used, provided significant improvement in literacy achievement of first-grade students. Flexer (2000) reported a study of three first-grade classrooms in Utah where 85% of the children were Native American. In the five years prior to sound field use, only 44% to 48% of first-grade children scored at the "basic" level and above on the Utah State Core Reading Test. After only seven months of sound field use, 74% of the fifty-four children in the study scored at the "basic" level and above. Another study found that phonemic awareness skills were most effectively and efficiently taught in preschool and kindergarten classrooms that had sound field distribution systems. In fact, the fewest at-risk readers came out of the classrooms that routinely used their sound field distribution systems (Flexer, Biley, Hinkley, Harkema, & Holcomb, 2002). These studies support the strong auditory basis of literacy. Clearly, the ability to discriminate word-sound distinctions impacts literacy development.

Understanding Sound Field Technology from a Universal Design Rather Than from a Treatment Perspective

Historically, amplification technologies such as hearing aids, personal FM systems, and now cochlear implants have been recommended as treatments for hearing loss. Because there certainly are populations for whom an enhanced signal-to-noise ratio can mean the difference between passing and failing in school, sound field technologies came to be recommended as treatments for hearing problems. If viewed as a treatment, sound field technology is recommended for a particular child and managed through the special education system.

However, with the recognition that all children require an enhanced signal-to-noise ratio comes the necessity of moving beyond thinking of sound field technology as a treatment. Sound field distribution systems need to be integrated into the general education arena. The concept of universal design can be useful in this regard.

The concept of universal design originated in the architectural domain with the common examples of curb cuts, ramps, and automatic doors. After years of use, modifications that were originally believed to be relevant for only a few people were discovered to be useful and beneficial for a large percentage of the population.

In terms of learning, universal design means that the assistive technology is not specially designed for an individual student but rather for a wide range of students. Universally designed approaches are implemented by general education teachers rather than by special education teachers ("Universal design," 1999). It is critical to note that implementation of sound field technologies is shifting from the special education to the general education arena.

Teacher In-Services: A Necessity for Effective Equipment Use

Difficulties with sound field technology can result from two primary categories: lack of teacher and administrator information about the rationale and use of the technology, and inappropriate setup and function of the equipment itself (Boothroyd, 2002). See Box 1-1 for a detailed outline of information to be presented during teacher in-services about the rationale and use of sound field systems.

Initial in-services to teachers and administrators need to emphasize the brain development purpose of acoustic accessibility. The relationship of hearing to literacy needs to be targeted, as does the fact that children listen differently than adults. The concept of signal-to-noise ratio needs to be explained. Microphone techniques need to be demonstrated to teachers so that they can learn how to use the equipment to teach incidental listening strategies. Teachers can use a much softer and more interesting voice because the sound field distribution system provides the vocal projection. Problems can result when teachers place limitations on their teaching or when they teach the same way with the technology as without it. A second microphone in the classroom—a pass-around microphone for the students (see Figure 1-2)—can greatly enhance teacher effectiveness. The pass-around microphone also allows children to hear each other, thereby increasing incidental learning and creating an auditory feedback loop through enhanced auditory self-monitoring of speech.

One point to emphasize when advocating for S/N ratio-enhancing technology is that acoustic accessibility is not a luxury—it is a necessity. Hearing is a first-order event for children in mainstreamed classrooms. If children cannot clearly and consistently hear classroom instruction, the entire premise of the educational system is undermined. Few families or schools have money for devices that are perceived as frills. However, when hearing takes its proper place at the head of the line relative to academic opportunities, then recommendations for S/N ratio-enhancing technologies are taken seriously.

Case Study Illustrating the Importance of Conducting In-Services

The educational audiologist and speech-language pathologist of a small city school district partnered with the local Quota Club (a club for professional women) to place infrared sound field systems in all kindergarten through

(case study continued on page 20)

> **Box 1-1   Rationale and Use of Sound Field Amplification: Outline for Teacher In-Service Training**

CONTENT AREAS

I. The World Has Changed
   A. Emphasis on literacy, including current statistics of pupils' reading performance
   B. Studies show that sound field amplification improves literacy
   C. The United States has a knowledge- and information-based economy

II. The Importance of Listening
   A. Hearing versus listening: auditory brain center access, stimulation, and growth
      1. Definition and differentiation of terms
      2. Sequential levels involved in auditory skill development
   B. Variables that affect listening
      1. Acoustic signal variables
      2. Listener response task variables
      3. Listening environment variables
      4. Listener-related variables: children do not listen like adults listen
      5. Speaker-related variables

III. Orientation to Sound and Its Properties
   A. Sound and sound waves
   B. Characteristics of sound
      1. Frequency
      2. Intensity
      3. Time
   C. Critical frequencies for speech perception
   D. Low- and high-frequency characteristics of speech sounds
   E. Activity: unfair spelling test

IV. Factors That Limit the Student's Ability to Listen
   A. Noise
   B. Reverberation
      1. Reverberation and reverberation time
      2. Effect of reverberation on speech perception
      3. Effect of age on speech perception under reverberant conditions

(continued)

Box 1-1 *(continued)*

  C. Effects of noise and reverberation on speech perception
      1. Synergistic phenomenon of noise and reverberation
      2. ANSI standards for classroom noise and reverberation levels
  D. Signal-to-noise (S/N) ratio, distance, and speech recognition
      1. Signal-to-noise (S/N) ratio
      2. Effect of S/N and distance on speech-recognition ability as a function of listener age

  V. Noise and reverberation sources
      A. External and adjacent classroom noise sources
      B. Internal classroom noise sources
      C. Common classroom noise levels
      D. Common environmental noise levels
      E. Reverberation sources

 VI. Materials and Strategies to Manage and Enhance Listening
      A. Noise and reverberation absorption materials
      B. Acoustical treatments
          1. External modifications
          2. Internal modifications
      C. Instructional strategies to improve classroom listening
      D. School-based noise reduction strategies

VII. Sound Field Amplification: FM and IR
      A. Orientation to sound field amplification
          1. Description of components, and distinguishing between FM and IR systems
          2. Demonstration of sound field amplification system
          3. Benefits of sound field amplification: FM and IR
          4. Factors to consider when recommending, purchasing, installing, and using sound field FM or IR amplification systems
      B. Transmitter and microphone options
          1. Options for wearing the transmitter or microphone
          2. Tips for successful use of the transmitter or microphone
          3. How to use the pass-around microphone for children
      C. Loudspeaker options
          1. Loudspeaker placement options
          2. Loudspeaker placement variables
      D. Setting the receiver or amplifier volume control

(continued)

Box 1-1 *(continued)*

    E. Sound field amplification system maintenance tips

    F. Sound field amplification system troubleshooting tips (wired system)

IN-SERVICE TRAINING MATERIALS

- Overhead projector
- Cassette tape player
- "Say What . . . ? An Introduction To Hearing Loss" (includes the unfair spelling test and can be obtained from the American Academy of Audiology, http://www.audiology.org)
- Sound-level meter
- Sound field amplification system—FM or IR—(installed) with available microphone options, including the second pass-around microphone
- Auxiliary input cords and adapters
- Participant notebooks (copies of transparencies and pertinent reference items such as troubleshooting and maintenance checklists, equipment and support literature from the manufacturer, and so on)

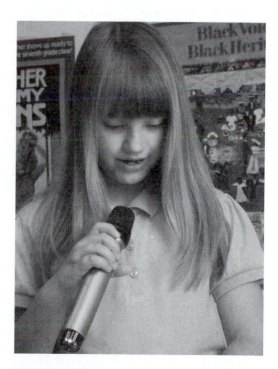

Figure 1-2: The pass-around microphone also allows children to hear each other, thereby increasing incidental learning and creating an auditory feedback loop through enhanced auditory self-monitoring of speech. (Photograph courtesy of LightSPEED Technologies.)

third-grade classrooms in the district. Prior to installation, I was invited to assist them in a district-wide teacher and administrator in-service. We followed the basic format discussed in this chapter and demonstrated the use of the sound system while giving our presentation. Most teachers and principals were very keen to use the systems. However, one longtime second-grade teacher was reluctant. She said that she had a loud voice and all could easily hear her. We explained that according to an analysis of acoustic phonetics, a loud voice indeed put more sound in the room—but ironically, the speech would be less clear due to upward spread of masking. That is, 90% of the energy of speech is in the low frequencies, but only 10% of the intelligibility resides there. Intelligibility (hearing word and sound distinctions) is carried by the weak high-frequency sounds. So, a loud voice powers the vowels but can obscure the consonants. Moreover, a loud voice can sound harsh and monotonous due to speaking at the edge of the vocal range. We encouraged her to try the sound field unit for two weeks and coached her to use a softer, more soothing voice. Let the equipment, not her, do the work of distributing the sound, we advised. Both the audiologist and speech-language pathologist visited her several times during the two-week trial to coach her in vocal use and the teaching of pupil-listening strategies. After two weeks' time, the teacher again met with us. She said, "I'm a believer!" She reported that she had overheard two of her students say that they were glad that their teacher wasn't mad anymore—she finally stopped yelling! The teacher went on to say that her class felt calmer and the students were more focused. Transition time between activities was reduced. In addition, the teacher said that she was amazed that she felt less fatigued in the evenings. As an aside, her principal told us that it was a joy not to hear that teacher's voice booming down the hallway. He was surprised that the teacher sounded much quieter when she used the sound system than when she did not.

This case study illustrates the importance of conducting teacher in-services prior to installation, augmented by follow-up coaching after installation. Besides providing critical information, in-services offer an opportunity for concerns to be expressed and for misconceptions to be clarified. Without an in-service, this second-grade teacher likely would not have used the sound system, and 28 children per year would have been denied acoustic accessibility!

SUMMARY

Key educational issues that typically have been ignored are the listening demands placed on children in poor acoustic environments, compounded by the immature listening skills that children bring to a classroom situation.

Hearing is a first-order event in a mainstream classroom. If a child cannot clearly hear spoken instruction, the entire premise of the educational system is undermined. Due to poor acoustic conditions and a variety of hearing and attending problems, there are millions of children who are being denied an appropriate education.

Sound distribution systems must be featured when discussing the classroom listening environment, because these systems improve the S/N ratio. The better and more consistent the S/N ratio, the more accessible will be the teacher's spoken instruction to the brains of pupils. Therefore, using a universal design paradigm, sound field technology ought to be included in general education classrooms and not be limited to special education on a case-by-case basis.

All that is at stake in this time of rapid change is the future of this country.

DISCUSSION TOPICS

1. Discuss how sound field technology and literacy development impact the future of this country.
2. How does an understanding of the levels of auditory skill development pertain to the need for sound distribution systems?
3. How can speech be heard as audible but still not be intelligible?
4. Identify key issues that need to be covered in teacher in-services.
5. Detail how children listen differently than adults.

REFERENCES

Alter, J. (1999, September 20). Bridging the digital divide. *Newsweek,* p. 55.

Anderson, K. L. (2001, April). Voicing concern about noisy classrooms. *Educational Leadership,* pp. 77–79.

Berg, F. S. (1993). *Acoustics and sound systems in schools.* Clifton Park, NY: Thomson Delmar Learning.

Berlin, C. I., & Weyand, T. G. (2003). *The brain and sensory plasticity: Language acquisition and hearing.* Clifton Park, NY: Thomson Delmar Learning.

Bess, F. H., & L. E. Humes (2003). *Audiology: The fundamentals* (3rd ed.). Philadelphia: Lippincott Williams & Wilkins.

Bhatnagar, S. C. (2002). *Neuroscience for the study of communicative disorders* (2nd ed.). Philadelphia: Lippincott Williams & Wilkins.

Boothroyd, A. (1997). Auditory development of the hearing child. *Scandinavian Audiology, 26*(Suppl. 46), 9–16.

Boothroyd, A. (2002). *Optimizing FM and sound-field amplification in the classroom.* Paper presented at the American Academy of Audiology National Convention, Philadelphia.

Chermak, G. D., & Musiek, F. E. (1997). *Central auditory processing disorders: New perspectives.* Clifton Park, NY: Thomson Delmar Learning.

Crandell, C., & Smaldino, J. (2002). *Classroom acoustics.* Paper presented at the American Academy of Audiology National Convention, Philadelphia.

Darai, B. (2000). Using sound field FM systems to improve literacy scores. *ADVANCE for Speech-Language Pathologists & Audiologists, 10*(27), 5, 13.

Erber, N. (1982). *Auditory training.* Washington, DC: The Alexander Graham Bell Association for the Deaf.

Flexer, C. (1989). Turn on sound: An odyssey of sound field amplification. *Educational Audiology Association Newsletter, 5,* 6–7.

Flexer, C. (1998). *Enhancing classrooms for listening, language, and literacy.* Videotape. Layton, UT: Info-Link Video Bulletin.

Flexer, C. (1999). *Facilitating hearing and listening in young children* (2nd ed.). Clifton Park, NY: Thomson Delmar Learning.

Flexer, C. (2000). The startling possibility of soundfield. *ADVANCE for Speech-Language Pathologists & Audiologists, 10,* 5, 13.

Flexer, C., Biley, K. K., Hinkley, A., Harkema, C., & Holcomb, J. (2002). Using sound-field systems to teach phonemic awareness to pre-schoolers. *The Hearing Journal, 55*(3), 38–44.

Johnson, S. (1998). *Who moved my cheese?* New York: G. P. Putnam's Sons.

Knittel, M. A. L., Myott, B., & McClain, H. (2002). Update from Oakland schools sound field team: IR vs FM. *Educational Audiology Review, 19*(2), 10–11.

Leavitt, R. J., & Flexer, C. (1991). Speech degradation as measured by the rapid speech transmission index (RASTI). *Ear and Hearing, 12,* 115–118.

Ling, D. (2002). *Speech and the hearing impaired child* (2nd ed.). Washington, DC: The Alexander Graham Bell Association for the Deaf and Hard of Hearing.

National Center for Education Statistics: National Assessment of Educational Progress (NAEP). (2001). *1992–2000 Reading Assessments.* Washington, DC: U.S. Department of Education, Office of Educational Research Improvement.

Niskar, A. S., Kieszak, S. M., Holmes, A., Esteban, E., Rubin, C., & Brody, D. F. (1998). Prevalence of hearing loss among children 6 to 19 years of age: The third national health and nutrition examination survey. *Journal of the American Medical Association, 279*(14), 1071–1075.

Robertson, L. (2000). *Literacy learning for children who are deaf or hard of hearing.* Washington, DC: The Alexander Graham Bell Association for the Deaf and Hard of Hearing.

Rosenberg, G. G., Blake-Rahter, P., Heavner, J., Allen, L., Redmond, B. M., Phillips, J., & Stigers, K. (1999). Improving classroom acoustics (ICA): A three-year FM sound field classroom amplification study. *Journal of Educational Audiology, 7,* 8–28.

Ross, M., Brackett, D., & Maxon, A. (1991). *Assessment and management of mainstreamed hearing-impaired children.* Austin, TX: Pro-Ed.

Sharma, A., Dorman, M. F., & Spahr, A. J. (2002). A sensitive period for the development of the central auditory system in children with cochlear implants: Implications for age of implantation. *Ear and Hearing, 23*(6), 532–539.

Sloutsky, V., & Napolitano, A. (2003, May–June). Auditory versus visual dominance in preschool children. *Child Development, 15–20.*

Trelease, J. (2001). *The read-aloud handbook* (5th ed.). New York: Penguin Books.

Universal design: Ensuring access to the general education curriculum. (1999). *Research Connections in Special Education, 5,* 1–2.

CHAPTER 2

Modeling the Effects of Room Acoustics on Speech Reception and Perception

Arthur Boothroyd, PhD

KEY POINTS

- The total speech signal at the listener's ear is a combination of the direct speech signal and the early components of reverberation.
- The total noise at the listener's ear is also a combination of two factors— the actual background noise and the late components of reverberation.
- At around eight feet, the direct speech signal and reverberation are equal, leading to a 3 dB increase in the total speech level. This distance is known as the critical distance.
- The amount of useful acoustic information available to a listener in a room is dependent on the effective signal and the effective noise. The effective signal-to-noise ratio is the difference between the total speech signal and the total noise level.
- The Speech Audibility Index can be used to estimate recognition of acoustic cues, speech segments, isolated words, and words in context. In order to most effectively increase the Speech Audibility Index, one must reduce background noise and the late components of reverberation.
- Acoustic conditions that produce acceptable levels of speech reception and perception for adults may be inadequate for children in a learning environment.
- Acoustic modification to the room, sound field systems, and personal FM amplification can improve the detrimental effects of signal-to-noise ratio and reverberation in rooms with less than ideal acoustics.

INTRODUCTION

Communication by spoken language involves a complex chain of events, as illustrated in Figure 2-1. A critical link in this chain is the effective transmission of sound from the talker's mouth to the listener's ear, which can be helped or hindered by the acoustical characteristics of the communication setting. The information on speech reception in this chapter can be used, within limits, to make predictions about the accuracy of speech perception. The mathematics that follow underlying the material are included for those readers who wish to explore the topic further. Other readers, however, may skip the boxes containing the math without losing the narrative flow.

NOISE AND REVERBERATION

Of the many factors that influence the quality of a room's acoustics, background noise and reverberation are the two most important.

Background Noise

Background noise is any sound that is unrelated to the speech of the talker. It can be generated in the room by other occupants or by equipment. It can also be generated outside the room, gaining access through air spaces; through walls, windows, ceilings, floors, and doors; or through the building's structure. High levels of background noise have the obvious effect of masking some of the important cues in the acoustic speech signal. Less obvious effects include listener distraction and listener fatigue. The talker may also experience fatigue, and even vocal abuse, in efforts to overcome excessive noise.

Reverberation

Reverberation is the persistence of sound in a room because of multiple reflections from its boundaries. Some energy is lost by absorption at each reflection, so the reverberant sound does not persist forever. Instead, it dies away gradually once the sound source stops. When measured in terms of sound energy, the decay of sound is exponential—that is, it falls rapidly at first but then more and more slowly as time progresses. When sound energy is converted to decibels, however, the rate of decay is constant in decibels per second.

Reverberation Time

Reverberation time is defined as the time taken for the sound level to fall by 60 dB, after the source is turned off. In large rooms, with lots of sound-reflect-

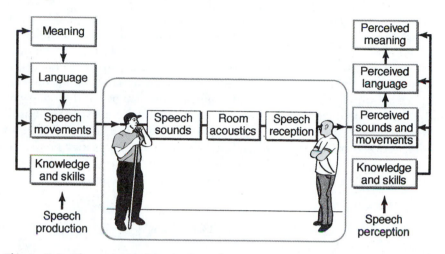

Figure 2-1. The acoustic properties of a room influence the integrity of the received speech signal during communication. Although spoken language communication is complicated and depends on numerous factors, the effective transmission of sound patters from talker to listener is critical.

ing surfaces (glass, concrete, chalkboards, ceramic tiles, etc.), several seconds may elapse before the level of the reverberant sound falls by 60 dB. In small rooms, with lots of sound-absorbing surfaces (rugs, curtains, upholstery, acoustic tiles, etc.), reverberation times are typically less than half a second. The occupants of a room also serve as sound absorbers. A room filled with people will usually have a lower reverberation time (by between one-twentieth and one-tenth of a second) than the same room unoccupied.

Early Components

Reverberation is not all bad. The early components of reverberation (also known as early reflections) reach the listener's ear soon enough that the listener's brain can ignore the delay and use them to enhance perception (Latham, 1979; Bradley, 1986a, 1986b; Bradley, Sato, & Picard, 2003). These early components of reverberation have usually undergone only a few reflections on the way to the listener's ear. Acoustic designers can often use early reflections as one way to enhance speech reception.

Late Components

The late components of reverberation, however, are destructive. They reach the listener's ear too late to be useful for perception of the speech sounds they represent. If loud enough, they may also interfere with the perception of subsequent speech sounds (Bradley, Sato, & Picard, 2003). They have usually undergone many reflections on their way to the listener's ear. Good acoustic design involves minimizing the late components of reverberation by judicious placement of sound-absorbing materials. Defining early and late in this context is not easy, because the distinction depends, in part, on the overall reverberation time and on the talker's speech characteristics. In general, however, reflections with delays of less than fifty milliseconds can be considered early, while those with delays in excess of one hundred milliseconds can be considered late. The crossover point, in the region of seventy-five milliseconds, is no coincidence; this point approximates the average duration of a single speech sound (vowel or consonant) in connected speech. Figure 2-2 gives a visual illustration of the difference between early and late reflections.

THE TOTAL SPEECH SIGNAL

The total speech signal at the listener's ear is a combination of the direct speech signal and the early components of reverberation. To determine the level of the combined signal, we need to know the levels of the separate contributions.

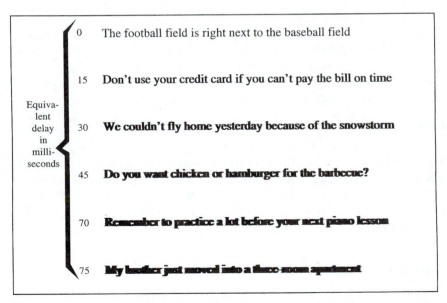

Figure 2-2. A visual analogy of the differential effects of early and late reflections on speech perception. Additional copies (reflections) of each sentence have been overlaid on the original but displaced (delayed) by increasing amounts. Short delays enhance perception, but long delays degrade it.

The Direct Speech Signal

The direct speech signal travels in a straight line from talker to listener without being involved in any reflections. Its level, however, falls by 6 dB for every doubling of distance from the talker. A typical long-term average speech level at one foot from the talker's mouth might be 72 dB SPL. This level will drop to 66 dB SPL at two feet, 60 dB SPL at four feet, 54 dB SPL at eight feet, and so on. For a child who is thirty-two feet from the teacher, the level of the direct speech signal would only be around 42 dB SPL. The equation relating received direct speech level to distance from the source is:

$$d = s - 20\log(f) \tag{2.1}$$

where d = level of direct speech in dB, s = level of original speech in dB at one foot and zero degrees azimuth, and f = distance from talker to listener in feet.

Early Components of Reverberation

The level of the early components of reverberation can be considered, to a first approximation, to be uniform throughout the room. This level depends on four factors: the speech output level and directionality of the talker, and the volume and reverberation time of the room.

Directionality (Q) refers to the tendency of a source to radiate sound energy in a forward direction rather than equally in all directions. The value of Q for a typical talker is around 4, in the frequency region of most importance to speech perception. This means that if the talker radiated speech as well in all directions as in the forward direction, the total energy sent into the room (in that frequency region) would be multiplied by a factor of 4. Directionality is one of the reasons that speech perception becomes more difficult when the talker's back is to the listener (Bradley, Sato, & Picard, 2003).

If the talker's voice rises by a certain number of decibels, the early components of reverberation will increase by the same amount. In addition, other things being equal, the level of the early reverberation will be higher when:

1. the room is small (hence the pleasure of singing in the shower),
2. the source is less directional, or
3. the room has a long reverberation time.

The equation relating the early components of reverberation to the four key variables is:

$$e = s - 10\log(vQ/r) \tag{2.2}$$

where e = level of early components of reverberation in dB, s = level of original speech in dB SPL at one foot and zero degrees azimuth, v = volume of room in cubic feet, Q = directionality of source, and r = reverberation time of room in milliseconds (see Davis & Davis, 1997).

Combining Direct Speech and Early Reverberation

To combine the direct speech signal with the early components of reverberation, we must first convert the decibel levels to energy units and add. We can then convert back to decibel levels. When the two levels are equal, addition results in a doubling of energy, or a 3 dB increase. If the levels differ by 10 dB or more, the level of the combination is, essentially, the level of the stronger component. The equation for decibel combination is:

$$TS = 10\log(10^{(d/10)} + 10^{(e/10)}) \tag{2.3}$$

where TS = total signal level in dB SPL, d = level of direct speech signal as developed in Equation 2.1, and e = level of early reverberation as defined in Equation 2.2.

Figure 2-3 shows predicted speech levels for a room with a reverberation time of 0.5 seconds, measuring $36 \times 24 \times 9$ feet, and a talker with a Q of 4, generating 72 dB SPL at 1 foot. Speech levels are shown as a function of distance from the talker. (The level of late reverberation is also shown, but this will be discussed later.) Note that close to the talker, the direct speech predominates, but far away reverberation predominates. At around 8 feet, the two are equal, leading to a 3 dB increase in the total speech level.

This distance is known as the *critical distance.* It is generally thought that beyond the critical distance, the direct speech signal can be ignored, but, in fact, one needs to be at least three times the critical distance from the talker before the direct signal makes negligible contribution, in this case at around 24 feet. The children in the last two rows of Figure 2-3, for example, are listening almost entirely to the early components of reverberation, which are at 54 dB SPL. Similarly, one needs to be less than one-third of the critical distance from the talker before reverberation makes negligible contribution, in this case less than 3 feet. The relevance of this last point to FM and/or sound field amplification should be obvious. Note, also, that the predictions in Figure 2-3 assume that the talker is facing the listener. If the talker's head turns, the level of the direct signal will fall and the critical distance will decrease (Bradley, Sato, & Picard, 2003). The level of the early reverberation, however, can be assumed to be unchanged.

THE TOTAL EFFECTIVE NOISE

The total noise at the listener's ear is also a combination of two factors: the actual background noise and the late components of reverberation.

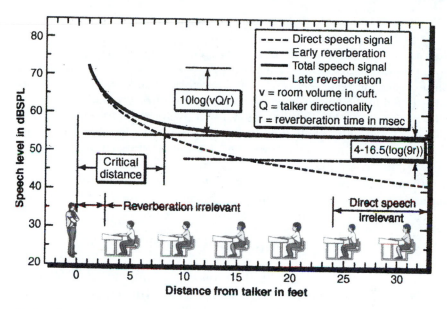

Figure 2-3. Received speech and reverberation levels for a room with a reverberation time of 0.5 seconds, measuring 36 × 24 × 9 feet. The talker level at 1 foot is assumed to be 72 dB, and talker Q is assumed to be 4. Note that the values of Q and r apply to the frequency region around 2 kHz, which is the most important frequency region for speech perception.

Actual Background Noise

As indicated earlier, the background noise is unrelated to the speech signal. Its level can take any value. Its spectral content and amplitude versus time envelope will depend in part on the sources and in part on the reverberant properties of the room. Ideal classrooms will have a background noise of less than 40 dBA (that is, 40 dB measured with the A setting of a sound-level meter, so as to weight different frequency regions according to the sensitivity of the human ear). However, rooms in which the background noise level is in excess of 55 dBA are very common (Picard & Bradley, 2001). Low frequencies tend to predominate in the spectrum of background noise, but this is not always the case. From the point of view of speech perception, noise in the frequencies around 2,000 Hz is the most damaging because these frequencies carry much of the most useful information in speech. Noise is subject to the effects of reverberation in the same way that speech is. In general, reverberation tends to increase noise level. It also tends to remove temporal gaps, or spaces, in the noise. These gaps have been shown to improve speech perception, at least for persons with normal hearing (Festen & Plomp, 1990). When measuring the level of background noise in a room, however, the effects of reverberation are already present and need not be accounted for further.

Late Components of Reverberation

Because the late components of reverberation interfere with speech perception, they can be treated as an equivalent noise. In essence, reverberation causes speech to generate its own masking noise. The average level of this noise is tied to the level of the early components of reverberation, which is directly tied to the level of the original speech signal. If, for example, the talker's voice rises by 10 dB, then both the early and the late components of reverberation will increase by 10 dB. The difference between the levels of the early and late components, however, depends on the reverberation time of the room. The lower the reverberation time, the greater the difference between the early and late components. The equation relating effective noise level to early reverberation and reverberation time is:

$$l = e - 16.5(4 - \log(9r)) \tag{2.4}$$

where l = effective noise level of late reverberation in dB SPL, e = level of the early reverberation as defined in Equation 2.2, and r = reverberation time in milliseconds. (Based on the work of Peutz, 1997.)

Figure 2-3 includes information on the late components of reverberation for the particular room and talker illustrated. In this example, the equivalent noise level of the late reverberation is around 48 dB SPL. This is only 6 dB below the level of the early reverberation. The children in the last three rows are, therefore, restricted to an effective signal-to-noise (S/N) ratio of only 6 or 7 dB, even if there is no significant background noise.

Combining Actual Noise and Late Reverberation

As with the total signal, we calculate the total noise level by converting the decibel levels of the actual background noise and the effective noise created by late reverberation to energy units, adding, and converting back to dB. The equation for combining actual background noise with the late components of reverberation is:

$$TN = 10\log(10^{(n/10)} + 10^{(l/10)}) \tag{2.5}$$

where TN = total noise level in dB SPL, n = level of actual noise in dB SPL, and l = effective noise created by late reverberation, as defined in Equation 2.4.

When the level of the actual background noise is 10 dB or more below that of the late reverberation, the contribution of background noise can be ignored. Similarly, if the level of the actual background noise is 10 dB or more above that of the late reverberation, then the contribution of reverberation can be ignored. These points are illustrated in Figure 2-4, which shows total

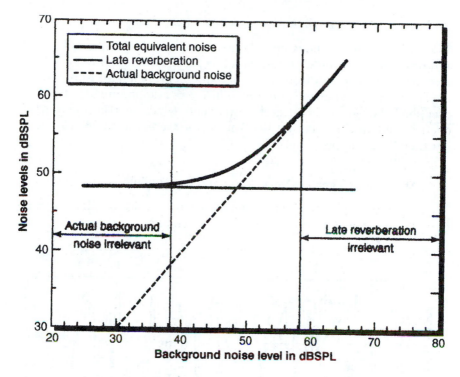

Figure 2-4. The result of combining actual background noise and the effective noise produced by the late components of reverberation for the room illustrated in Figure 2–3.

noise level as a function of actual background noise level for the room illustrated in Figure 2-3. As Figure 2-4 illustrates, there is little to be gained by lowering background noise below 38 dB SPL.

EFFECTIVE SIGNAL-TO-NOISE RATIO

Having defined the total speech signal and the total noise level, we are now in a position to define the effective signal-to-noise ratio as the difference between the two.

$$ESN = TS - TN \tag{2.6}$$

where ESN = effective signal-to-noise ratio in dB, TS = total speech level in dB SPL as defined by Equation 2.3, and TN = total noise level in dB SPL as defined by Equation 2.5.

Variation of Speech Level over Time

So far, we have been dealing with the long-term average levels of speech, noise, and reverberation. The short-term level of the acoustic speech signal, however, varies considerably from moment to moment. When measured over a time interval of around one hundred milliseconds (approximating the time over which the human ear integrates sound energy), the level in any given frequency band varies from about 15 dB above the average to 15 dB below it, as illustrated in the upper panel of Figure 2-5.

Short-Term Signal-to-Noise Ratio and the Audibility of Speech

Assume, for the moment, that the total noise has no short-term level fluctuations. Because the short-term speech level is fluctuating over a range of 30 dB,

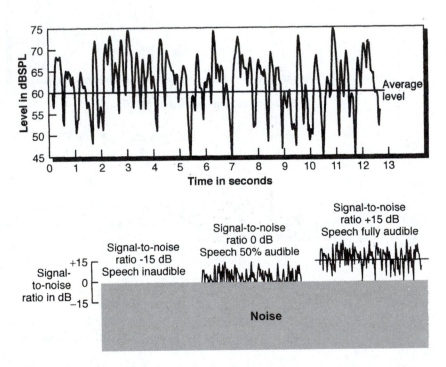

Figure 2-5. The upper panel shows the variation of short-term speech level (measured over 100 msec intervals) as a function of time for a woman speaking a series of sentences. Note that short-term level varies from around 15 dB above to 15 dB below the long-term average level. The lower panel illustrates how the signal rises from inaudible to fully audible as the signal-to-noise ratio rises from –15 dB to +15 dB.

the short-term signal-to-noise ratio also varies over a range of 30 dB, from 15 dB above its average value to 15 dB below it. Furthermore, the average signal level needs to be at least 15 dB above the average noise level in each frequency band if the useful speech information in that band is to be fully audible. Similarly, the average speech level would need to be at least 15 dB *below* the average noise level in order for the speech in that band to be fully masked by the noise. Halfway between, when the average speech and noise levels are the same, roughly 50% of the useful speech information would be audible. In other words, the speech signal in a given frequency band rises from inaudible to fully audible as the effective signal-to-noise ratio in that band rises from −15 dB to +15 dB. These points are illustrated in the lower panel of Figure 2-5. Even if the noise level has short-term fluctuations, the basic conclusions still hold.

SPEECH AUDIBILITY INDEX

The foregoing considerations lead to the concept of a Speech Audibility Index.

Definition

Speech Audibility Index is here defined as the percentage of the useful acoustic signal in the combined direct speech and early reverberation whose level exceeds that of the combined background noise and late reverberation.

Speech Audibility Index cannot be lower than 0% or higher than 100%. Between these limits, its value rises uniformly from 0% to 100% as the effective signal-to-noise ratio rises from −15 dB to +15 dB. The equation relating Speech Audibility Index to signal-to-noise ratio is:

$$SAI = (ESN + 15)/30*100 \qquad (2.7)$$

where SAI = Speech Audibility Index in %, with limits of 0% and 100%, and ESN = effective signal-to-noise ratio in dB as defined by Equation 2.6.

Multi- versus Single-Band Implementation

The models developed so far allow for the conversion of information about talker speech level, talker directionality, talker distance, room volume, background noise level, and reverberation time into an estimate of the audibility of the useful information in the acoustic speech signal. A complete implementation of this model requires its application to multiple frequency bands and the integration of the results based on the relative importance of those bands. If a single-band implementation is required, this can be based on an octave band centered around 2,000 Hz. This band contains some of the most useful information in the acoustic speech signal. One can also use a single-band implementation if the signal-to-noise ratio is independent of frequency—that is, if the noise and the speech have the same long-term average spectrum.

Relationship to Other Audibility Indices

Speech Audibility Index is derived using the basic principles of Articulation Index theory (French & Steinberg, 1947; Fletcher, 1953; American National Standards Institute, 1995). Articulation Index (AI) and its more recent instantiation, Speech Intelligibility Index (SII) (American National Standards Institute, 2002a), do not, however, account for the negative effects of the late components of reverberation. Speech Transmission Index (STI) and its abbreviated version, Rapid Speech Transmission Index (RASTI), do account for reverberation (Steeneken & Houtgast, 1973). STI can be considered interchangeable with Speech Audibility Index when applied to room acoustics. Speech Transmission Index, however, is defined in terms of the influence of noise and reverberation on variations of amplitude envelope over time, and it must be measured at multiple locations in a room with equipment that is specially designed for the purpose. In contrast, the room data required for estimating Speech Audibility Index at a particular location (i.e., background noise level and reverberation time) can be obtained with a general-purpose sound-level meter. If the sound-level meter does not include the capability for measuring reverberation time, this can be estimated from the areas and sound absorption properties of the surfaces in the room. And if the background noise is uniformly distributed, the effects of distance from the source can be estimated from the models developed in this chapter, thereby avoiding the need to make measurements at multiple locations. In spite of their differences, the goal of all these indices is the same—namely, to estimate from physical data, without resorting to behavioral measures of speech perception, the proportion of the useful information in the speech signal that is available at the listener's ear. It is important to remember, however, that Speech Audibility Index, and the other indices just mentioned, are estimates of speech *reception*. They are not estimates of speech *perception*. The extent to which speech reception estimates can be converted into speech-perception estimates is explored in the next section.

PREDICTING SPEECH PERCEPTION FROM SPEECH AUDIBILITY INDEX

Several problems are encountered when trying to convert Speech Audibility Index into estimates of speech-perception performance. One problem is that speech perception can be specified at many levels. Examples include acoustic cue perception, phoneme recognition in nonsense syllables, phoneme recognition in meaningful words, closed-set word identification, open-set word recognition, and word recognition in sentence context. A second problem is that at each of these levels, performance depends not only on the integrity of the sound patterns received by the listener but also on contextual evidence within and around the message, on the listener's knowledge and skills (a point emphasized in Figure 2-1), on the listener's auditory status, and on the properties of any sensory assistance. The following analyses are based on data from young adults with normal hearing and language. Probability theory is used first to predict the perception of acoustic cues from Speech Audibility Index. Predictions of phoneme and word recognition are then developed using two types of relationships that have been validated in previous work. The first relates the recognition of wholes to that of parts within wholes (for example, the recognition of words to that of phonemes within words). Key to this relationship is the j-factor, which is the effective number of independent parts that must be recognized in order to recognize the whole. The second type of relationship deals with the recognition of items with and without context (for example, recognition of words in sentences and words in isolation). Key to this relationship is the k-factor, which is the proportional increase in the effective number of independent channels of information introduced by the context (Boothroyd, 1978, 1985; Boothroyd & Nittrouer, 1988; Nittrouer & Boothroyd, 1990).

Acoustic Cue Perception

On the assumption that the evidence about acoustic speech cues is uniformly distributed across the 30 dB range of the speech signal, we can predict the probability of acoustic cue perception. This probability rises from 0% to almost 100% as Speech Audibility Index rises from 0% to 100%. Recognition probability and Speech Audibility Index are not equal, however, because of redundancy in the speech signal. In fact, when only half of the useful information is available to the listener, the probability of correctly perceiving acoustic speech cues is close to 90%. Note that the probability of perceiving acoustic speech cues never quite reaches 100%, even when the speech signal is fully audible. There is always a finite probability of error. In normally hearing adults, this probability appears to be around 0.7%, or 0.007. This residual error will probably be higher in young children; listeners with deficits of hearing, language, attention, or processing; and listeners to a nonnative language. The equation predicting acoustic cue perception from Speech Audibility Index is:

$$ac = 100(1 - (re/100)^{(SAI/100)}) \qquad (2.8)$$

where ac = recognition probability for acoustic cues in %, SAI = Speech Audibility Index in %, and re = residual error in %, when SAI = 100% (= 0.7% for hearing adults).

Phoneme Recognition in Consonant-Vowel-Consonant Words

The recognition of phonemes normally requires the accurate perception of more than one acoustic cue. Empirical data indicates that young adults require, on average, the accurate perception of around two independent acoustic cues per phoneme (Boothroyd & Guerrero, 1996). In addition, the placement of phonemes in meaningful consonant-vowel-consonant words has been shown to increase the effective number of channels of independent information in young hearing adults by a factor of 1.3 (Boothroyd & Nittrouer, 1988). The equation predicting phoneme recognition from acoustic cue perception is:

$$ph = 100(1 - (1 - (ac/100)^{j1})^{k1}$$ (2.9)

where ac = probability of acoustic cue perception as defined in Equation 2.8, $j1$ = average number of independent acoustic cues per phoneme (= around 2.0 for young hearing adults), and $k1$ = the influence of word context on phoneme recognition (around 1.3 for young hearing adults).

These factors can be taken into account in order to predict phoneme recognition probability (in meaningful consonant-vowel-consonant words) from Speech Audibility Index. Figure 2-6 shows the results together with empirical data obtained from young normally hearing adults (Boothroyd & Guerrero, 1996). Note that the number of independent acoustic cues per phoneme will most likely be higher in young children; listeners with deficits of hearing, language, attention, or processing; and listeners to a nonnative language. We have no evidence, however, to suggest that the benefits of word context for children as young as five years old are less than those for young adults, providing the words are within their vocabulary (Nittrouer & Boothroyd, 1990).

Recognition of Whole Consonant-Vowel-Consonant Words

When measuring speech perception using consonant-vowel-consonant words, there are two scoring options. The clinician or researcher can measure either the percentage of whole words correct or the percentage of the constituent phonemes correct. The two performance measures are not identical, but they are related by a j-factor, which is a measure of the effective number of independent phonemes that need to be recognized, on average, in order for a whole word to be recognized (Boothroyd, 1985; Boothroyd & Nittrouer,

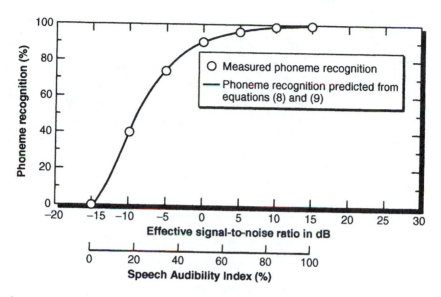

Figure 2-6. Measured and predicted phoneme recognition in consonant-vowel-consonant words as a function of effective signal-to-noise ratio and Speech Audibility Index. The data points are means for eight young, normally hearing adults listening to consonant-vowel-consonant words in a steady state noise whose spectrum was matched to that of the talker. The line is a least-squares fit to Equations 2.8 and 2.9.

1988). In nonsense syllables or unfamiliar words, j equals the number of actual phonemes per word (three in the case of consonant-vowel-consonant words). In meaningful consonant-vowel-consonant words, j for young adults is typically in the region of 2.5. The equation predicting consonant-vowel-consonant (CVC) word recognition from phoneme recognition is:

$$w = 100(ph/100)^{j2} \qquad (2.10)$$

where w = word-recognition probability in %; ph = phoneme recognition probability in %, as defined in Equations 2.8 and 2.9; and $j2$ = average number of independent phonemes per CVC word (= around 2.5 for young hearing adults and randomly chosen words).

Figure 2-7 shows predicted whole word recognition as a function of signal-to-noise ratio for j-factors of 1.0, 2.0, and 3.0. Note that the use of very easy or common words would tend to lower the value of j, toward 2.0. However, the value of j will be closer to 3.0 in young children; listeners with deficits of hearing, language, attention, or processing; and listeners to a nonnative language.

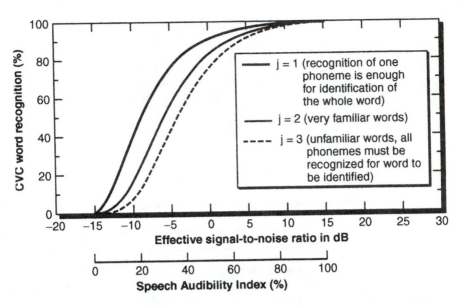

Figure 2-7. Predicted consonant-vowel-consonant word recognition as a function of effective signal-to-noise ratio and Speech Audibility Index. Predictions are based on Equations 2.8, 2.9, and 2.10 and are shown for three values of the j-factor.

Recognition of Words in Sentences

Placement of words in sentence context increases their probability of recognition (Miller, Heise, & Lichten, 1955). The presence of sentence context is equivalent to multiplying, by a k-factor, the number of independent channels of information that are available for perception of the individual words. In nonsense sentences, where the context is of no help, the k-factor equals 1.0. In complex sentences with low predictability, the k-factor might be around 2.0. In simple sentences with high predictability, however, the k-factor can be 10 or more. In other words, in casual conversation between adults, the context can be contributing 10 times as much information as the actual acoustic speech signals. For a given type of sentence material, the k-factor will lower for young children; listeners with deficits of hearing, language, attention, or processing; and listeners to a nonnative language. Figure 2-8 shows predicted word-in-sentence recognition probability as a function of signal-to-noise ratio for values of k ranging from 1 to 16. Note that the k-factor is assumed to be independent of signal-to-noise ratio in Equation 2.11 and Figure 2-8. Research has shown, however, that the k-factor tends to increase under difficult listening conditions as listeners begin to rely more on the sentence context and less on the degraded acoustic signal (Grant & Seitz, 2000; Boothroyd, 2002).

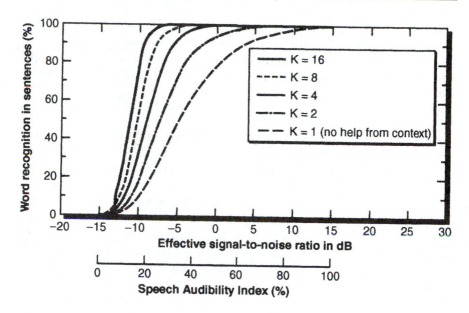

Figure 2-8. Predicted word recognition in sentences as a function of effective signal-to-noise ratio and Speech Audibility Index. Predictions are based on Equations 2.8–2.10 and are shown for values of the k-factor ranging from 1 (each word in the sentence must be recognized on its own merits, as if heard in isolation) to 16 (easy, highly predictable sentences).

The equation predicting word recognition in sentence context from word recognition in isolation is:

$$ws = 100 \; (1 - (1 - (wi/100))^{k2}) \qquad (2.11)$$

where ws = word-recognition probability in sentences; wi = word-recognition probability in isolation, as defined in Equations 2.8, 2.9, and 2.10; and $k2$ = effective proportional increase in number of independent channels of information provided by the sentence context.

Figure 2-8 illustrates an important fact about the relationship between room acoustics and speech perception. Levels of noise or reverberation that might be considered acceptable for one type of speech material, perceptual task, or listener can be totally unacceptable for others. Consider, for example, the perception of words in highly predictable sentences such as might be used in casual conversation. Assume that the appropriate k-factor is 8. Figure 2-8 predicts that word recognition under this condition would approach 100% at an effective signal-to-noise ratio of –5 dB. But to achieve the same recognition probability for isolated consonant-vowel-consonant words would require a signal-to-noise ratio of +15 dB even for adults. Clearly, acoustic conditions that might be considered appropriate for casual conversation between adults can be entirely inadequate for children in a learning environment, where much of the spoken language involves difficult material containing unfamiliar vocabulary.

SPEECH AUDIBILITY INDEX AND SPEECH PERCEPTION IN A ROOM

We are now in a position to recreate Figure 2-3 in terms of the model developed above and embodied in the various equations. Figure 2-9 shows the predicted values of Speech Audibility Index, word recognition in isolation and word recognition in difficult (k = 2) and easy (k = 8) sentences. The various parameters are based on empirical data from young adults with normal hearing and language who are listening in their native language. In the upper left panel, the background noise (35 dB SPL) is well below the level of the late components of reverberation. This room meets the recently promulgated ANSI standard for new or renovated classrooms (American National Standards Institute, 2002b). Listening conditions are excellent throughout the room with the possibility of a few errors of isolated word recognition for individuals who are farthest from the talker.

The lower left panel of Figure 2-9 illustrates the effects of introducing high levels of background noise. Word recognition in easy sentences remains high, even at considerable distance from the talker. But word recognition in difficult sentences falls to unacceptably low levels (except, perhaps, for the individual in the first row, and even that individual has difficulty with words in isolation). Similar conclusions would be reached for the upper right panel of Figure 2-9, which illustrates the effect of increasing reverberation time to 1.5 seconds while maintaining a low noise level. Finally, the lower right panel of Figure 2-9 shows the combined effect of high noise and high reverberation. Now, even the perception of easy sentences is compromised except, perhaps, for the individuals in the first two rows.

Note, again, that the predictions illustrated in Figure 2-9 are based on data from young adults with normal hearing and language. Speech-perception performance would be expected to be poorer for young children; listeners with deficits of hearing, language, attention, or processing; and listeners to a nonnative language (Neuman & Hochberg, 1983; American Speech-Language-Hearing Association, 1995; Johnson, 2000). Our field is badly in need of empirical data on the quantitative effects of noise, reverberation, distance, and message redundancy on spoken language perception in these populations.

On the positive side, the model developed here takes no account of the potential benefits of binaural hearing (Neuman & Hochberg, 1983) and the

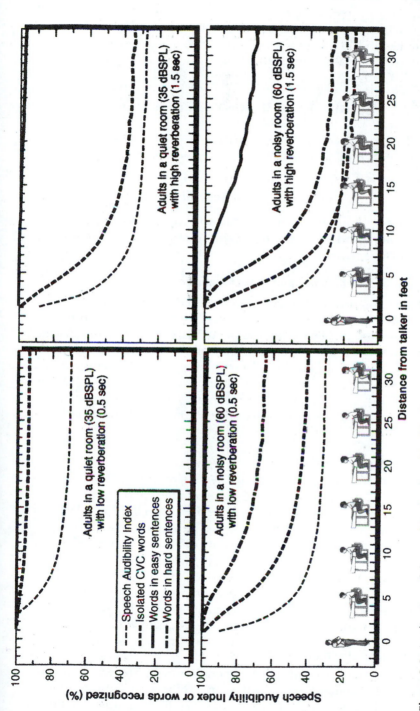

Figure 2-9. Application of the models developed in this chapter to the prediction of speech reception (Speech Audibility Index) and speech perception (word recognition), as functions of distance, for the room illustrated in Figure 2–3. The top left panel shows predictions for the original conditions of low noise and low reverberation. The effects of high noise, high reverberation, and both are illustrated in the other three panels. The model parameters used here are based on data from young adults with normal hearing.

integration of hearing and speech-reading, both of which can enhance perception under difficult listening conditions. Once again, however, there is a pressing need for research data on these effects in real classrooms.

ENHANCING SPEECH RECEPTION

The models developed in this chapter have implications for methods used to improve speech reception in classrooms and other listening spaces.

Improving Room Acoustics

The most obvious approach to increasing Speech Audibility Index is to reduce background noise and the late components of reverberation (Crandell & Smaldino, 2000).

Need to Consider Both Noise and Reverberation

Dealing with only noise or only reverberation, however, may not be enough. There is little point in reducing noise if reverberation is the primary problem, or in reducing reverberation if noise is the primary problem. Consider the room illustrated in Figures 2-3 and 2-4, for example. Efforts to reduce background noise below 38 dB SPL will have negligible payoff unless reverberation time is also reduced. Consider also the illustrations in Figure 2-9. If we take the noisy reverberant room (bottom right) and control only noise (top right), the benefits are limited. The same is true if we control only reverberation (bottom left). Maximum benefit occurs when both are controlled (top left).

Need to Preserve Early Reflections

When working to minimize the late components of reverberation, it is important to remember that these efforts will also reduce the level of the early components. This, in turn, will lower the total received speech level for listeners who are far from the talker. In a large classroom with good acoustic treatment, for example, listeners in the back row may have difficulty hearing the teacher simply because the received speech level is too low in relation to listeners' threshold of hearing or to background noise (see Figure 2-3). Efforts to reduce reverberation should not be overdone. An appropriate compromise must be found between the need to reduce the late components of reverberation and the need to preserve the early components (Bradley, Sato, & Picard, 2003).

Enhancing Early Reflections

Although the levels of early and late reverberation are tied together, enhancing the early reflections in relation to the late reverberation is possible, up to a point. This is done by the judicious placement of reflecting surfaces between talker and listener. In this connection, note that the common practice of covering the entire ceiling with acoustic tiles can deprive listeners of one of the primary sources of early reflections (American National Standards Institute, 2002b).

Need for Appropriate Expertise

The basic methods for reducing internally generated noise, keeping out externally generated noise, and controlling reverberation are well understood. Their proper implementation in the design or modification of real rooms, however, requires considerable expertise, typically found in acoustical engineers and acoustical consultants. Audiologists can play a valuable role in identifying and quantifying bad acoustics and in specifying desirable goals for their improvement. When it comes to the specifics of how those goals will be met, however, the involvement of someone with the appropriate training and experience is important.

Sound Field Amplification

Bringing Speech Audibility Index to acceptable levels throughout an intended listening area by acoustic treatment alone is not always possible. Limiting factors can include cost, uncontrollable noise sources, overriding concerns about air quality or temperature, and loss of early reflections. In such situations, there may be much to be gained by sound field amplification (also known as sound reinforcement). The talker's speech is picked up by a microphone placed a few inches from the lips, and the resulting signal—free of noise and reverberation—is delivered at an appropriate level to one or more strategically placed loudspeakers.

Dealing with Distance and Noise

The benefits of sound field amplification are most obvious when the primary limitations are distance and noise. Under these conditions, the total speech level can be increased at the listener's ear while the total noise level remains unchanged. The resulting improvement of signal-to-noise ratio has an immediate effect on Speech Audibility Index—at the rate of just over three percentage points for every decibel increase (see Equation 2.7). Three factors can influence the actual benefit: the number of loudspeakers, the effective gain of the system, and proximity of the listener to a loudspeaker. Consider, for example, the situation in which the effective gain of the system is zero. That is, the speech output level of each loudspeaker (measured at, say, three feet) is equal to that of the person wearing the microphone (also measured at three feet, even though the microphone is at only a few inches). Assume also that the directionality of the talker and the loudspeakers are the same. If only a single loudspeaker is used, the total energy in the direct and early reflected signals will be doubled, resulting in a 3 dB increase of signal level for listeners who are more than three times the critical distance from both sources. The resulting increase in signal-to-noise ratio for these students translates into a 10 percentage point increase in Speech Audibility Index. We can increase the benefit further by increasing the number of loudspeakers, increasing the output of each loudspeaker (by turning up the volume control of the amplifier or moving the microphone closer to the talker's mouth), placing loudspeakers closer to the listeners, or some combination of these. (See Chapter 8 for additional discussion of sound field speakers.)

Dealing with Reverberation

When the primary problem in a room is the level of late reverberation, sound field amplification must be selected and installed with great care. Any increase in level of the direct and early reflected signals that comes from increasing the number of loudspeakers, or the system gain, causes an equal increase in the level of late reverberation. As a result, Speech Audibility Index for listeners who are far from the talker or one of the loudspeakers remains constant and, in extreme cases, may actually fall. To a certain extent, this problem can be dealt with by taking advantage of two of the variables that affect reverberation—directionality and proximity. By using speakers with high directionality and placing them as close to the listeners as possible, we can provide a high effective signal-to-noise ratio for the maximum number of listeners. Care must be taken, however, to maintain uniform coverage and to avoid problems of acoustic feedback. In reverberant rooms, the quality of the sound field system and the expertise of the designers and installers become of primary importance.

Importance of Preserving High Frequencies

When a sound field system begins to howl because of acoustic feedback, using the tone control to reduce amplification of the higher frequencies is tempting. Unfortunately, this is a poor solution. Although the low-frequency gain preserves the loudness of the amplified signal (Cox & Moore, 1988; Boothroyd, Erickson, & Medwetsky, 1994), the loss of high-frequency gain deprives the listeners of those frequencies that are most important to the perception of speech (French & Steinberg, 1947). If acoustic feedback becomes a problem, it should be solved by changes of loudspeaker placement or reduction of overall system gain. It should not be solved by reducing high-frequency gain alone.

Limitation

An important characteristic of sound field amplification is that it only provides improved reception for the speech of the person wearing the microphone. To the extent that learning in a particular classroom involves each student hearing the comments, questions, and answers of other students, this characteristic may be a limitation. A teacher who is aware of the problem, however, can deal with it by developing appropriate compensatory strategies. Examples include passing the microphone to a student who has something to say and repeating the contributions of students.

Personal FM Amplification

The most extreme way to take advantage of proximity is to transmit the signal from a close-talking wireless microphone directly to the hearing aid or cochlear implant of a hearing-impaired listener, to a low-power hearing aid worn by a child with a processing or attention disorder, or to a small loudspeaker on the desk of any listener. Of all the techniques available for addressing problems of room acoustics, the personal FM system is by far the most effective (Ross, 1992). When using a sound field system, some of the negative effects of distance, noise, and late reverberation are reintroduced once the otherwise ideal signal emerges from the loudspeakers. In contrast, when using a personal FM system, the noise- and reverberation-free signal picked up by the microphone is preserved at the ear of the listener. As with the sound field system, however, the benefit of personal FM applies only to the speech of the person wearing the microphone. Note, also, that simultaneous activation of both the remote wireless microphone and a hearing aid's (or cochlear implant's) own microphone can negate the FM benefit unless the gains via the two microphones are carefully adjusted in relation to each other (American Speech-Language-Hearing Association, 2002).

SUMMARY

Effective reception of the acoustic speech signal is central to communication by spoken language. The effective signal received by a listener in a room is a combination of the direct speech signal, traveling in a straight line without reflection, and the early components of reverberation. The value of the effective signal is diminished, however, by the effective noise, which is a combination of actual noise and an equivalent noise generated by the late components of reverberation. The effective signal-to-noise ratio is the difference, in decibels, between the effective signal and the effective noise. Speech Audibility Index is a measure of how much of the useful information in the signal is available to the listener. It rises from 0% to 100% as the effective signal-to-noise ratio rises from −15dB to +15 dB. Speech Audibility Index can be used to estimate the recognition of acoustic cues, speech segments, isolated words, and words in sentence context. Converting from speech reception to speech perception, however, introduces nonacoustic variables. These variables include the nature and complexity of the language and the auditory status, language status, knowledge, and skill of the listener. Acoustic conditions that guarantee a suitable level of speech reception and perception for adults listening to informal conversation may be totally inadequate for children in a learning situation, especially if those children have deficits of hearing, language, attention, or learning or if they are listening in a nonnative language. Optimizing Speech Audibility Index requires coordinated control of both background noise and reverberation. Sound field and personal FM amplification can reduce the negative effects of distance, noise, and reverberation in rooms with less-than-ideal acoustics, at least for the speech of the person wearing the microphone.

DISCUSSION TOPICS

1. Describe the effects of reverberation, including both early and late components.
2. From the point of view of speech perception, which frequencies are the most damaging? Why?
3. What are the conditions in which background noise can be ignored?
4. Explain the problems that are encountered when trying to convert Speech Audibility Index into estimates of speech-perception performance.
5. Explain how one could increase Speech Audibility Index by reducing background noise and the late components of reverberation.
6. When and how might one utilize sound field amplification to bring Speech Audibility Index to acceptable levels?

REFERENCES

American National Standards Institute. (1995). *American national standard method for measuring the intelligibility of speech over communications systems* (ANSI S3.2–1989, R 1995). New York: Author.

American National Standards Institute. (2002a). *American national standard methods of the calculation of the speech intelligibility index* (ANSI S3.5–1997, R 2002). New York: Author.

American National Standards Institute. (2002b). *Acoustical performance criteria, design requirements, and guidelines for classrooms* (ANSI S12.6–2002). New York: Author.

American Speech-Language-Hearing Association. (1995, March). Acoustics in educational settings: Position statement and guidelines. *ASHA, 37*(Suppl. 14), 15–19.

American Speech-Language-Hearing Association. (2002). Guidelines for fitting and monitoring FM systems. *ASHA Desk Reference* (Vol. II, pp. 151–171). Rockville, MD: Author.

Boothroyd, A. (1978). Speech perception and sensorineural hearing loss. In M. Ross & G. Giolas (Eds.), *Auditory management of the hearing-impaired child.* Baltimore: University Park Press.

Boothroyd, A. (1985). Evaluation of speech production in the hearing-impaired: Some benefits of forced-choice testing. *Journal of Speech and Hearing Research, 28,* 185–196.

Boothroyd, A. (2002). Influence of context on the perception of spoken language. In *Proc. Congreso Internacional de Foniatra, Audiologa, Logopedia y Psicologa del lenguaje.* Universidad Pontificia de Salamanca.

Boothroyd, A., Erickson, F., & Medwetsky, L. (1994). The hearing aid input: A phonemic approach to assessing the spectral distribution of speech. *Ear and Hearing, 15,* 432–442.

Boothroyd, A., & Guerrero, N. (1996). *Normal performance vs. intensity functions for CASPA.* Unpublished report, City University of New York.

Boothroyd, A., & Nittrouer, S. (1988). Mathematical treatment of context effects in phoneme and word recognition. *Journal of the Acoustical Society of America, 84,* 101–114.

Bradley, J. S. (1986a). Predictors of speech intelligibility in rooms. *Journal of the Acoustical Society of America, 80,* 837–845.

Bradley, J. S. (1986b). Speech intelligibility studies in classrooms. *Journal of the Acoustical Society of America, 80,* 846–854.

Bradley, J. S., Sato, H., & Picard, M. (2003). On the importance of early reflections for speech in rooms. *Journal of the Acoustical Society of America, 113,* 3233–3244.

Cox, R. M., & Moore, J. R. (1988). Composite speech spectrum for hearing aid gain prescriptions. *Journal of Speech and Hearing Research, 31,* 102–107.

Crandell, C. C., & Smaldino, J. J. (2000). Classroom acoustics for children with normal hearing and with hearing impairment. *Language, Speech, and Hearing Services in Schools, 31,* 362–370.

Davis, D., & Davis, C. (1997). *Sound system engineering* (2nd ed.). Newton, MA: Focal Press.

Festen, J. M., & Plomp, R. (1990). Effects of fluctuating noise and interfering speech on the speech-reception threshold for impaired and normal hearing. *Journal of the Acoustical Society of America, 88,* 1725–1736.

Fletcher, H. (1953). *Speech and hearing in communication.* New York: Van Nostrand. (Available in the ASA edition, edited by Jont Allen and published by the Acoustical Society of America in 1995.)

French, N. R., & Steinberg, J. C. (1947). Factors governing the intelligibility of speech sounds. *Journal of the Acoustical Society of America, 19,* 90–119.

Grant, K. W., & Seitz, P. F. (2000). The recognition of isolated words and words in sentences: Individual variability in the use of sentence context. *Journal of the Acoustical Society of America, 107,* 1000–1011.

Johnson, C. E. (2000). Children's phoneme identification in reverberation and noise. *Journal of Speech, Language, and Hearing Research, 43*(1), 144–157.

Latham, H. G. (1979). The signal-to-noise ratio for speech intelligibility: An auditorium acoustics design index. *Applied Acoustics, 12,* 253–320.

Miller, G. A., Heise, G. A., & Lichten, W. (1955). The intelligibility of speech as a function of the context of the test material. *Journal of Experimental Psychology, 41,* 329–335.

Neuman, A. C., & Hochberg, I. (1983). Children's perception of speech in reverberation. *Journal of the Acoustical Society of America, 73*(6), 2145–2149.

Nittrouer, S., & Boothroyd, A. (1990). Context effects in phoneme and word recognition by young children and older adults. *Journal of the Acoustical Society of America, 87,* 2705–2715.

Peutz, V. (1997). Speech recognition and information. Appendix 10 in Davis, D., & Davis, C. (1997). *Sound system engineering* (2nd ed., pp. 639–644). Newton, MA: Focal Press.

Picard, M., & Bradley, J. S. (2001). Revisiting speech interference in classrooms. *Audiology, 40*(5), 221–244.

Ross, M. (Ed). 1992. *FM auditory training systems.* Timonium, MD: York Press.

Steeneken, H. J. M., & Houtgast, T. (1973). The modulation transfer function in room acoustics as a predictor of speech intelligibility, *Acustica, 28,* 66–73.

ACKNOWLEDGMENT

Preparation of this chapter was supported by grant H1343E980010 from the National Institute of Disability Rehabilitation and Research (NIDRR) to the Rehabilitation Engineering Research Center at Gallaudet University.

CHAPTER 3

Speech Perception in the Classroom

Joseph J. Smaldino, PhD

Carl C. Crandell, PhD

KEY POINTS

- The primary goal of the classroom educational process is to share experiences, exchange ideas, and transmit knowledge.
- Accurate transmission of acoustic information and adequate knowledge of language are important determinants of speech perception.
- For accurate speech perception to occur, stored knowledge bases must exist and be intact.
- The knowledge bases are developmental and become more complete and refined with experience.
- In the beginning of the language-learning process, acoustic information is often novel and requires analytic processing via a mode called serial processing.
- Serial processing is a slower mode and requires a great deal of cognitive energy to attend to and establish linkages to the knowledge bases.
- As language develops, the acoustic signal can be processed in a less cognitively demanding mode called parallel processing.
- It is important to determine where speech perceptual breakdowns in individual students occur and to intervene to overcome these deficits.

The majority of this book is devoted to a discussion of acoustic variables, such as signal-to-noise (S/N) ratio and reverberation in the classroom. Indeed, the impact of these acoustic factors on a student's ability to perceive spoken language is our main thesis. In order to understand the impact of acoustic variables and the basis for acoustic management and habilitative intervention, a simple model of the speech perceptual process may be helpful to the reader. Using the model, we examine how the speech-perceptual competency that a student brings into the classroom is an important variable that determines how well he or she can use acoustic speech information and attain teacher understanding.

Certainly, the primary goal of the classroom educational process is to share experiences, exchange ideas, and transmit knowledge. This is accomplished by students not only because they are able to receive specific acoustic information, but also because they are able to relate these often ambiguous acoustic cues within the context of a language structure and to use circumstantial cues (Denes & Pinson, 1993).

SPEECH-PERCEPTION MODEL

A simplified model of speech perception is shown in Figure 3-1. The central thesis of this model is that incoming and stored knowledge interact to result in accurate speech perception. Distortions of incoming information or incomplete stored knowledge can impair a student's ability to perceive the speech information so critical to success in school. Let us examine how incoming and stored information interact differently to produce accurate and faulty speech perception.

In order for accurate speech perception to occur, stored knowledge bases must exist and be intact. The knowledge bases are developmental and become more complete and refined with experience. Normal principles of language acquisition operate to guide the induction of an acoustic/linguistic language system (McCormick & Schiefelbusch, 1984; Sanders, 1993; McLaughlin, 1998). As shown in Figure 3-1, an acoustic signal, containing acoustic cues critical to speech perception, attracts the attention of the developing language processing system. In the beginning of the language-learning process, much of this acoustic information is novel and requires close scrutiny. The signal is analytically processed in a mode called serial processing. It is during serial processing that speech and language acoustic patterns are analyzed, structured, and stored. A real-world example of serial processing might be when one first attempts to learn a foreign language. Most of the new language elements are novel and must be broken down into individual sounds; rules for linking words must be studied, and vocabulary must be learned. Because so much analysis is needed, processing of utterances in the new language is slow. When an individual is first learning a new language, native speakers seem to be speaking at unrealistically fast rates. The truth is that the native speakers are not speaking at a fast rate; the new learner of the language is processing the speech at a slow rate!

When in the serial processing mode, one's ability to understand what is being said is greatly influenced by distortions of the incoming signal—such as background noise, reverberation, reduced visual cues, and fast-speaker rate—

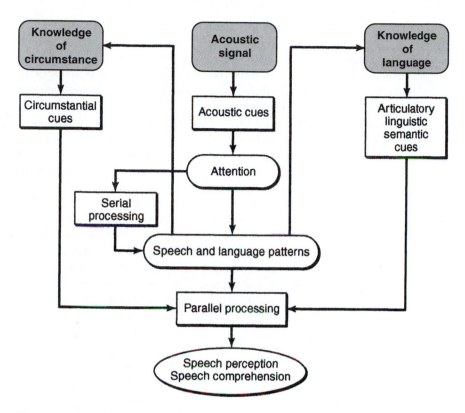

Figure 3-1. Simplified model of speech perception.

because the advantages of being able to predict distorted or incomplete speech comes with a developed knowledge of the language. Eventually, the acoustic patterns are linked to articulatory movements and linguistic/semantic rules. In addition, circumstantial cues such as identity of the speaker and visual information are also tied to the patterns. All of these rules and cues work together to duplicate and constrain the possible interpretation of the incoming signal. This acquisition system is so efficient that once it is formed, another more efficient form of attentional processing can be used. With so much duplication and constraint on the incoming signal, the signal no longer needs to be dissected in order to be understood; it can now be synthetically processed in larger chunks in a less cognitively demanding mode called parallel processing. Going back to our real-world example, parallel processing becomes dominant after a listener becomes familiar with a foreign language, when accurate perception occurs rapidly and effortlessly. Native speakers no longer seem to be speed-talkers, and the listener can keep up with the message they are transmitting. Distortion of speech does not affect understanding as drastically as in the serial processing mode because a more developed language knowledge allows the listener to predict speech based on incomplete acoustic information. Normal speech perception can be thought of as such a process. While the quality of the incoming acoustic signal is an important variable for accurate speech perception in the classroom, circumstantial cues and the status of the student's knowledge about the language are also significant variables.

Inaccurate speech perception can occur because of a breakdown in any of the aforementioned variables. Let us take each variable and describe possible effects from the model in Figure 3-1. The acoustic speech signal contains cues to accurate speech perception. If there is a hearing loss, even a slight hearing loss, some of these cues will be attenuated, filtered, or distorted. Poor classroom acoustics can have the same effect on the incoming signal and have similar effects on the speech-processing model. Let us assume that an incoming signal is distorted in frequency, intensity, and time domains. The novel signal will be attended to by the student, and serial processing will occur. As part of this processing mode, linkages to the other knowledge bases will be made. In a very young child, these distorted signals will form the knowledge bases, and as a consequence they will be incomplete. There is no need to dwell on the well-known faulty language systems that develop in most severely hearing-impaired children without intervention (Boothroyd, 1984; Sanders, 1993). However, subtle abnormalities in language linkage will occur even if the distortion to the incoming signal is slight. In older children who have normally established language linkages, distortion can make an incoming signal novel, that is, different from expectation based on already established language linkages. In either case, the child may be forced into a serial processing mode—an analytical mode—in an attempt to reconcile the discrepancies between the incoming signal and the language knowledge base. As noted before, serial processing is a slower mode and requires a great deal of cognitive energy to attend to and try to establish linkages to the knowledge bases. Often, children in this mode cannot keep up with the speed of the incoming signal and need more time to reconcile it to what they know. Remember the example of beginning to learn a foreign language. Becoming lost in the incoming information flow, the child may only receive fragments of the signal or lose attentiveness and process unimportant parts of the signal. The parallel processing mode is never fully engaged. Further degradation of the incoming signal due to noise or other distortion makes the situation worse because the child has little reliable redundant information to fall back on. Such is faulty speech perception.

So far, this chapter has demonstrated that the analysis, structure, and storing of the incoming signal necessary for speech perception is a multivariable process. Speech perception is dependent not only on receipt of specific acoustic information, but also on the student's ability to relate these often ambiguous cues within the context of a language structure and circumstantial cues.

Breakdowns in the system produce faulty speech perception. Much of this book is devoted to breakdowns in the incoming acoustic signal, but in this chapter our focus is on breakdowns in the language system that can impair integration of the incoming acoustic signal into a language context and can produce faulty perception as well. Auditory health care professionals, who justifiably focus on the integrity of the incoming acoustic signal, often minimize the possibility that even in the presence of a complete acoustic signal, faulty speech perception can occur. Under these circumstances, repair of a faulty incoming acoustic signal alone may not improve speech perception. The purpose of the next section is not to review the research in detail or debate theoretical issues concerning different models of speech perception or mechanisms of language acquisition; see Ferrand (2001) and McLaughlin (1998) for a discussion of these issues. Instead, the intent is to provide a sense of the variables that can impair a student's ability to analyze and perceive the spoken word in the classroom.

LEARNING STRATEGIES

Returning to the model in Figure 3-1, speech perception is dependent on receipt of specific acoustic information and also on the ability to relate these often ambiguous cues within the context of a language structure and circumstantial cues. The cognitive activities that tie the acoustic signal to language are referred to as learning strategies (McCormick & Schiefelbusch, 1984). Breakdowns in the processes underlying the cognitive activities will impair the tie between the acoustic signal and language and thus produce faulty perception. In the model shown in Figure 3-1, cognitive activities are represented by the boxes labeled "attention," "speech and language patterns," "serial processing," and "parallel processing."

Attention

The ability to focus selectively on relevant features of an incoming acoustic signal is developmental. As the overall speech perceptual system matures, attention becomes more and more selective, and preferences or biases are established (Gibson, 1969). In the classroom, the ability to sustain focus is also very important. McCormick and Schiefelbusch (1984) refer to sustained attention as attention span, or on-task behavior. Educators relate the amount of time that a student is on task to success in learning (Cangelosi, 1991). Students who are unable to attend selectively to a signal or who cannot maintain sustained attention (such as those with attention deficit disorder) have a roadblock in the speech perceptual model shown in Figure 3-1. In the case of unselective attention, irrelevant signals will be as equally accessible to the speech perceptual process as are relevant signals. The student may focus on noise and distractions rather than on important speech signals. One need only think of the unselective attention of the autistic child to demonstrate the outcome of this kind of cognitive inability. Delight in the hum of a refrigerator motor while totally disregarding relevant commands is all too familiar to the parents of an autistic child (Lovaas & Schreibman, 1979). How relevant analysis of speech can occur under these circumstances is difficult to imagine. The inability to sustain attention or stay on task can also block perception. Feagans, Sanyal, Henderson, Collier, and Applebaum (1987) hypothesized that the long-term effect of reduced hearing might well be that the student learns to become inattentive to language. Analysis of the incoming acoustic speech signal requires sustained attention, especially if the serial processing mode is in use. Ironically, the student with the weakest ability to analyze language might well require the greatest attentional ability. Fortunately, selective attention and sustained attention appear to be skills that can be taught if difficulties in these areas are recognized early (Gibson, 1969; Feagans et al., 1987).

Concept Formation

The details of concept formation in the language-learning process are well beyond the scope of this chapter; Bloom and Lahey (1978) offer a full discussion of the establishment of linguistic and nonlinguistic concepts. However, as should be clear from the model in Figure 3-1, a great deal of mental activity is involved in establishing speech and language patterns, in serial and parallel processing, and in the establishment of relationships between linguistic and nonlinguistic signals and meaning. A breakdown in concept formation affects perception because the manner and efficiency with which sensory information is organized determines to a large extent how useful it will be for future reference (McCormick & Schiefelbusch, 1984).

Storage and Retrieval

Speech perception is accomplished by combining incoming acoustic signals with stored knowledge about language and knowledge of the context or circumstance of the communicative message. Thus, speech perception is the result of an interaction between incoming and stored information (Denes & Pinson, 1993). A detailed discussion of the mechanisms that have been theorized for storage and retrieval of information in the nervous system are outside the scope of this chapter; for more information on these theories, see Geis and Hall (1977), Kobashigawa (1976), and McCormick and Schiefelbusch (1984). Whatever the memory process, incoming information must be organized in a manner that allows efficient storage and quick retrieval. The retrieved information must be in a form that can be combined with incoming information and derived perceptions. Needless to say, considerable cognitive ability is required to accomplish these tasks in real time. Breakdowns in the storage or retrieval process can have devastating effects on speech perception. One need only consider the communicative plight of the receptive or expressive aphasic person to understand the consequences in the extreme. Less severe breakdowns can slow the speech-processing system down and impair the listener's ability to store and retrieve information in real time. Becoming lost in the incoming information stream most assuredly impairs speech perception.

The intent of this section was to provide a sense of the variables, besides the incoming acoustic signal, that can impair classroom speech perception. Selective and sustained attention abilities, competency in concept formation, and adequacy of storage and retrieval of information will not often be directly measured in children in the classroom. Most of these abilities can be inferred from competency in the use of language exhibited by the children. Children showing signs of language problems are in need of clinical intervention in order to maximize the use of the acoustic signal. If language problems are ignored, efforts to improve the incoming acoustic signal may not produce the expected improvements in classroom understanding.

SUMMARY

As was pointed out in the beginning of this chapter, the primary goal of the classroom educational process is to share experiences, exchange ideas, and transmit knowledge. This is accomplished by the students not only because they are able to receive specific acoustic information, but also because they are able to relate these often ambiguous cues within the context of a language structure and to use circumstantial cues. Not all acoustic information is specific enough and not all student speech perceptual systems are complete enough to allow the educational process to occur uninterrupted. The professional should identify and improve acoustic ambiguities caused by the classroom environment. Equally important are determining any speech perceptual breakdowns individual students may have, identifying who must interact with the acoustic signal in the classroom, and intervening clinically where possible. These steps, taken together, create a very good chance for strengthening the classroom educational process and improving student academic achievement.

DISCUSSION TOPICS

1. What other real-world examples might be used to depict the differences between serial and parallel speech processing?
2. In what ways do reverberation and background noise interfere with the development of an accurate knowledge base for a language?

3. In what ways are a clear acoustic signal and speech perceptual competency related to student academic achievement?

REFERENCES

Bloom, L., & Lahey, M. (1978). *Language development and language disorders.* New York: John Wiley & Sons.

Boothroyd, A. (1984). *Hearing impairments in young children.* Englewood Cliffs, NJ: Prentice-Hall.

Cangelosi, J. (1991). *Evaluating classroom instruction.* New York: Longman.

Denes, P. B., & Pinson, E. N. (1993). *The speech chain.* New York: W. H. Freeman & Company.

Feagans, L., Sanyal, M., Henderson, F., Collier, A., & Appelbaum, M. (1987). Relationship of middle ear disease in childhood to later narrative and attentional skills. *Journal of Pediatric Psychology, 12*(4), 581–594.

Ferrand, C. (2001). *Speech science.* Boston: Allyn & Bacon.

Geis, M., & Hall, D. (1977). Encoding and incidental memory in children. *Journal of Experimental Child Psychology, 22,* 58–66.

Gibson, E. (1969). *Principles of perceptual learning and development.* New York: Appleton-Century-Crofts.

Kobashigawa, A. (1976). Retrieval strategies in the development of memory. In R. V. Kail & J. W. Hagan (Eds.), *Memory in cognitive development.* Hillsdale, NJ: Lawrence Erlbaum Associates.

Lovaas, O., & Schreibman, L. (1979). Stimulus overselectivity in autism: A review of research. *Psychological Bulletin, 86,* 1236–1254.

McCormick, L., & Schiefelbusch, R. (1984). *Early language intervention.* Columbus, OH: Merrill Publishing.

McLaughlin, S. (1998). *Introduction to language development.* Clifton Park, NY: Thomson Delmar Learning.

Sanders, D. (1993). *Management of hearing handicap.* Englewood Cliffs, NJ: Prentice-Hall.

CHAPTER 4

Speech Perception in Specific Populations

Carl C. Crandell, PhD
Joseph J. Smaldino, PhD
Carol Flexer, PhD

KEY POINTS

- There are a number of populations of children with normal hearing sensitivity who experience significant difficulties understanding noisy or reverberated speech.
- These listeners include children with fluctuating conductive hearing loss, learning disabilities, articulation disorders, auditory processing deficits, language disorders, minimal degrees of sensorineural hearing loss (pure-tone sensitivity from 15 to 25 dB HL), unilateral hearing loss, and developmental delays and children for whom English is a second language.
- Acoustical criteria for appropriate noise levels and reverberation times have not been well established for these diverse populations of normal-hearing children.
- Until additional research is conducted, a conservative standard for noise levels and reverberation times in listening environments for normal-hearing children should follow the same acoustical recommendations utilized for listeners with hearing loss.

Listeners with sensorineural hearing loss (SNHL) are well recognized as experiencing greater difficulty understanding speech in noise or reverberation than normal hearers experience. What is not as well recognized is that there are a number of populations of children with normal hearing sensitivity who also experience significant difficulties understanding noisy or reverberated speech. As illustrated in Table 4-1, these listeners include children with fluctuating conductive hearing loss, learning disabilities, articulation disorders, auditory processing deficits, language disorders, minimal degrees of sensorineural hearing loss (pure-tone sensitivity from 15 to 25 dB HL), unilateral hearing loss, and developmental delays and children for whom English is a second language (Crandell & Smaldino, 1995a, 1995b). At present, the auditory, linguistic, and cognitive mechanisms responsible for perceptual difficulties in these populations remain unclear. This chapter will examine the effects of commonly reported classroom acoustics on the speech perception of children with SNHL as well as children with normal hearing. The next chapter in this book will address the influence of sound field amplification on the perceptual abilities and psychoeducational development of these populations.

CHILDREN WITH SENSORINEURAL HEARING LOSS

Recent estimates suggest that more than ten million school-age children exhibit some degree of SNHL. As discussed in previous chapters, children with SNHL require considerably better acoustical environments than do normal hearers in order to process and understand speech. Recall that children with SNHL require sound-to-noise (S/N) ratios surpassing +15 dB and reverberation times (RTs) no longer than 0.4 second for maximum communicative efficiency. Table 4-2 presents an illustration of the effects of hearing impairment on speech perception. These data, taken from Finitzo-Hieber and

---

TABLE 4-1   Populations of "normal hearing" children

- Young children (< 15 years old)
- Conductive hearing loss
- History of recurrent otitis media
- Language disorder
- Articulation disorder
- Dyslexia or other reading disorders
- Learning disabilities
- Nonnative English
- Auditory processing deficit
- Minimal degree of bilateral sensorineural hearing loss
- Unilateral sensorineural hearing loss
- Developmental delays
- Attentional deficits

Source: Table adapted from Crandell, Smaldino, and Flexer (1995).

TABLE 4-2   Mean speech-recognition scores (% correct) by children with normal hearing (N = 12) and children with sensorineural hearing loss (N = 12) for monosyllabic words across various S/N ratios and reverberation times (RT)

	Groups	
Testing Condition	**Normal Hearing**	**Hearing Impaired**
RT = 0.0 Seconds		
Quiet	94.5%	83.0%
+12 dB	89.2%	70.0%
+ 6 dB	79.7%	59.5%
0 dB	60.2%	39.0%
RT = 0.4 Seconds		
Quiet	92.5%	74.0%
+12 dB	82.8%	60.2%
+ 6 dB	71.3%	52.2%
0 dB	47.7%	27.8%
RT = 1.2 Seconds		
Quiet	76.5%	45.0%
+12 dB	68.8%	41.2%
+ 6 dB	54.2%	27.0%
0 dB	29.7%	11.2%

Source: Table adapted from Finitzo-Hieber and Tillman (1978).

Tillman (1978), show the speech-perception abilities of children (eight to twelve years of age) with mild to moderate degrees of SNHL (with and without amplification) compared to children with normal hearing sensitivity. Speech perception was assessed with monosyllabic words under various S/N ratios (quiet, +12, +6, 0) and reverberation times (RT = 0.0, 0.4, and 1.2 seconds). Results from this investigation reveal several trends. First, these data indicate that the children with hearing impairment performed significantly poorer than did the children with normal hearing across most listening conditions. Second, the performance decrement between the two groups increased as the listening environment became less favorable. For example, in what would be an extremely good classroom environment (S/N ratio = +12 dB; RT = 0.4 second), children with hearing impairment obtained speech-perception scores of only 60% compared to 83% for the normal hearers (a 13% difference). In acoustical conditions more commonly reported in the classroom (S/N ratio = +6 dB; RT = 1.2 seconds), the performance difference increased to 27%, with the children having SNHL obtaining speech-perception scores of just 27%.

CHILDREN WITH MINIMAL SENSORINEURAL HEARING LOSS

Despite the importance of providing an appropriate acoustic environment for children with SNHL, there remains a paucity of data concerning the communicative efficiency of children with minimal, or borderline, degrees of SNHL—that is, children with pure-tone thresholds between 15 and 30 dB HL through the speech-frequency range. Although the incidence of minimal hearing impairment in children is not exactly known, it is well recognized that incidence rates increase as a function of decreasing hearing loss (Bess, 1985; Bess & McConnell, 1981; Crandell, 1993a; Davis, Elfenbein, Schum, & Bentler, 1986). Therefore, it is reasonable to assume that a significant number of school-age children may exhibit minimal degrees of SNHL. Bess, Dodd-Murphy, and Parker (1998) reported that the incidence of minimal hearing loss was 5.4% in a sample of 1,218 school-age children. If this incidence rate was applied to all school-age children in the United States, this would suggest that approximately 2.5 million children exhibit minimal degrees of hearing loss. Overall, 37% of the children with minimal hearing loss had failed at least one grade. Moreover, children with minimal hearing loss exhibited higher degrees of psychosocial/physical health dysfunction in the areas of energy, behavior, stress, self-esteem, and social support as measured via the Dartmouth Primary Care Cooperative Information Project (COOP) Charts for Adolescents (Nelson, Wasson, Johnson, & Hays, 1996).

At present, few investigations have examined the effects of noise or reverberation on minimally hearing-impaired children. Boney and Bess (1984) demonstrated that children with minimal degrees of sensorineural hearing loss (pure-tone thresholds from 15 to 30 dB and from 500 to 2,000 Hz) experienced greater difficulty understanding speech degraded by noise and reverberation than did children with normal hearing sensitivity. Specifically, word- and sentence-recognition scores were obtained in four listening conditions: (1) quiet; (2) reverberation (RT = 0.8 second); (3) noise (S/N ratio = +6 dB); and (4) noise and reverberation (S/N ratio = +6 dB; RT = 0.8 second). Word-recognition results from this investigation indicated that the children with minimal hearing loss performed poorer than the control group, particularly in the degraded listening conditions.

Crandell (1993a) examined the speech perception of children with minimal degrees of sensorineural hearing loss at commonly reported classroom S/N ratios of +6, +3, 0, −3, and −6 dB. The children with minimal hearing loss exhibited pure-tone averages (0.5–2 kHz) from 15 to 25 dB HL. Speech perception was assessed with the Bamford-Koval-Bench (BKB) Standard Sentence test. Multitalker babble from the Speech Perception in Noise (SPIN) test was used as the noise competition. Mean sentence recognition scores (in % correct) as a function of S/N ratio are presented in Figure 4-1. Trends from these data are similar to those reported in children with greater degrees of SNHL. That is, children with minimal degrees of hearing impairment performed poorer than normal hearers across most listening conditions. Moreover, note that the differences in recognition scores between the two groups increased as the listening environment become more adverse. For example, at an S/N ratio of +6 dB, both groups obtained recognition scores in excess of 80%. At an S/N ratio of –6 dB, however, the minimally hearing-impaired group was able to obtain less than 50% correct recognition compared to approximately 75% recognition ability for the normal hearers.

Johnson, Stein, Broadway, and Markwalter (1996) evaluated speech perception in twelve young adults with normal hearing, twelve children with

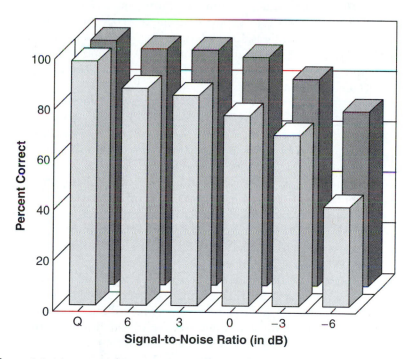

Figure 4-1. Mean speech-recognition scores (in % correct) of children with normal hearing (dark shaded bars) and children with minimal degrees of sensorineural hearing loss (light shaded bars) in quiet and at various signal-to-noise (S/N) ratios (SNRs). Figure adapted from Crandell, Smaldino, and Flexer (1995).

normal hearing, and twelve children with minimal degrees of high-frequency SNHL. Speech perception was assessed with nonsense syllables that were recorded in an average-sized classroom that had an RT of 0.7 second. Nonsense syllables were presented in quiet and in noise (S/N ratio = +13 dB). Results indicated that the children with minimal high-frequency SNHL obtained significantly poorer speech-perception scores in quiet when compared to children and adults with normal hearing. Surprisingly, the groups did not differ in speech-perception ability in noise. Certainly, the speech-perception difficulties experienced by children with minimal hearing loss may explain, in part, the psychoeducational and psychosocial deficits often seen in this population (Bess, 1985; Bess et al., 1998).

CHILDREN WITH NORMAL HEARING SENSITIVITY

Another group that exhibits speech-perceptual difficulties in the classroom is younger children with normal hearing sensitivity. Specifically, investigators have demonstrated that younger listeners require better acoustical environments than do adult listeners to achieve equivalent recognition scores (Crandell, 1992, 1993a, 1993b; Elliott, 1979; Elliott, 1982; Elliott et al. 1979; Nabelek & Nabelek, 1985). Adultlike performance on speech-perception tasks in noise or reverberation is generally not reached until the child reaches approximately thirteen to fifteen years of age.

Based on these data, it is reasonable to assume that commonly reported levels of classroom noise and reverberation could adversely affect the speech perception of younger children with normal hearing sensitivity. To support this assumption, the reader is again directed to the Finitzo-Hieber and Tillman (1978) data (see Table 4-2). Note that in typical classroom listening environments, the children with normal hearing generally obtained poor speech-perception scores. For example, in a relatively good classroom listening environment (S/N ratio = +6 dB; RT = 0.4 second), these children were able to recognize only 71% of the stimuli. In a poor but commonly reported classroom environment (S/N ratio = 0 dB; RT = 1.2 second), speech-perception scores were reduced to approximately 30%.

Crandell and Bess (1986) examined the speech perception of young children (five to seven years old) with normal hearing in a typical classroom environment (S/N ratio = +6 dB; RT = 0.45 second). Phonetically-Balanced Kindergarten (PBK) monosyllabic words were recorded through the Knowles Electronic Manikin for Acoustical Research (KEMAR) at speaker-listener distances often encountered in the classroom (6, 12, and 24 feet). Results from this investigation are presented in Figure 4-2. As can be noted, there was a systematic decrease in speech-perception ability as speaker-listener distance increased. Specifically, mean word-recognition scores of 89%, 55%, and 36% were obtained at 6, 12, and 24 feet, respectively. Overall, these results suggest

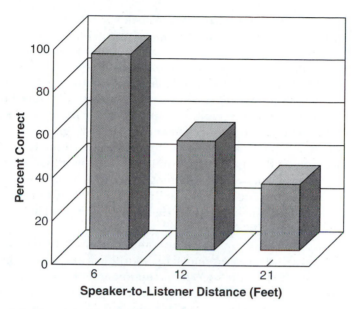

Figure 4-2. Mean speech-recognition scores (in % correct) of children with normal hearing in a typical classroom environment (S/N ratio = +6 dB; RT = 0.6 second) as a function of speaker-to-listener distance. Figure adapted from Crandell, Smaldino, and Flexer (1995).

that normal-hearing children seated in the middle to rear of a typical classroom setting have greater difficulty understanding speech than has traditionally been suspected.

These findings are understandable by examining those of a study by Leavitt and Flexer (1991). In this investigation, the authors utilized the Rapid Speech Transmission Index (RASTI) to estimate speech perception in a classroom. RASTI measurements are based on the hypothesis that noise and reverberation in a room will affect a speechlike signal in ways that can be related to speech perception. Results indicated that in a front-row center seat of the classroom, only 83% of the speech energy was available to the listener. Only 55% of the sound energy was available to the listener in the back-row center seat. Clearly, if only a fraction of the speech signal is available to the listener, poor speech perception will result.

CHILDREN FOR WHOM ENGLISH IS A SECOND LANGUAGE

Adult listeners for whom English is a second language often experience greater speech-perception difficulties than do native English listeners, particularly in degraded listening environments (Bergman, 1980; Crandell, 1991,

1992; Crandell & Smaldino, 1995a, 1995b; Nabelek & Nabelek, 1985). Bergman (1980), for example, examined the speech perception of adult native Hebraic listeners under various conditions of acoustic degradations, including noise (S/N ratio = +3 dB), reverberation (RT = 2.5 seconds), and split-band dichotic listening. Results indicated that the nonnative English subjects obtained significantly poorer perception scores than did the native English listeners across all listening conditions. Interestingly, these results were obtained although the native Hebraic listeners had been English speakers for more than fifty years. Such findings have important educational and therapeutic implications for the more than two million nonnative English children who may be exposed to unfavorable listening conditions in the classroom or resource-room environment (Crandell & Bess, 1986, 1987; Crandell, 1991, 1992, 1993a; Crandell & Smaldino, 1992, 1995a, 1995b; Finitzo-Hieber, 1988, Olsen, 1981, 1988; Ross, 1978).

Few investigations have examined the communicative efficiency of nonnative English-speaking children under real-world learning environments. Crandell (1996) examined the speech-perception abilities of twenty native English-speaking children and twenty nonnative English-speaking children under commonly reported classroom S/N ratios (+6 dB, +3 dB, 0 dB, –3 dB, –6 dB). Sentence recognition was assessed by BKB sentences, while the SPIN multibabble was used as the noise competition. Results from this investigation are shown in Figure 4-3. Although both groups obtained equivalent sentence-recognition scores in quiet, the nonnative English group performed significantly poorer at S/N ratios ranging from +3 to –6 dB.

CHILDREN WITH DEVELOPMENTAL DISABILITIES

Children with developmental disabilities are another population that would benefit, for a number of reasons, from the use of sound field amplification systems. First, attention to and concentration on tasks, which are basic requirements for learning, usually are deficient in special education populations. Second, there is a greater incidence of conductive hearing impairment among children who experience developmental disabilities than would be expected in a regular classroom population.

Flexer, Millin, and Brown (1990) conducted a study to determine if sound field amplification could reduce the effects of distractibility, conductive hearing loss, and typical levels of classroom noise in a class for students with developmental disabilities. Several conclusions were drawn from this investigation. First, the nine children who attended a primary-level class for students with developmental disabilities made significantly fewer errors on a word identification task when the teacher presented the words through the sound field amplification system than when the words were presented without amplification. Second, observation showed the children to be more relaxed and to

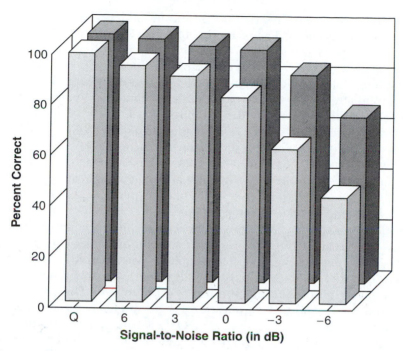

Figure 4-3. Mean speech-recognition scores (in % correct) of native English children (dark shaded bars) and nonnative English children (light shaded bars) in quiet and at various signal-to-noise (S/N) ratios. Figure adapted from Crandell, Smaldino, and Flexer (1995).

respond more quickly in the amplified condition. Third, only one of the nine children in the study had normal hearing (15 dB or better at all frequencies in both ears) and normal middle ear function when tested. The incidence of mild hearing impairment among special populations may be underestimated. Even though none of the children in the study was identified as hearing impaired according to generally accepted criteria, their minimal to mild hearing losses would interfere with classroom performance.

CHILDREN WITH CONDUCTIVE HEARING LOSS/RECURRENT OTITIS MEDIA

Approximately 76% to 95% of all children experience at least one episode of otitis media with effusion (OME) by six years of age. Additionally, 33% of all children develop persistent, or recurrent, OME during their first three years of life, a vital time for speech and language development. Although mild conductive hearing losses of 20–30 dB HL are common because of OME, hearing losses as great as 55 dB may be seen in some children (Bess & McConnell,

1981). Even mild losses of hearing can drastically influence the transmission of acoustical information. For example, Dobie and Berlin (1979) examined the potential loss of acoustical information in listeners with simulated losses of only 20 dB. Data indicated that children with mild degrees of conductive hearing loss would experience significant difficulty understanding brief utterances or high-frequency stimuli, particularly in degraded listening environments. In addition, these children would lose a majority of transitional information, such as final position consonants and plural endings. Recall that this loss of high-frequency acoustical information would be significant as research suggests that more than 90% of our understanding ability is derived from such phonemes. Discouragingly, research suggests that approximately 10–15% of all elementary school children are experiencing mild hearing losses associated with OME at any given time.

Crandell and Flannagan (1999) examined the effects of conductive hearing loss (CHL) caused by OME on speech perception. Subjects consisted of adults with normal hearing. Speech perception was assessed via the Modified Rhyme Test (MRT), while multitalker babble served as the noise competition. All stimuli was presented in quiet and at an S/N ratio of 0 dB. The speech stimuli was presented at normal conversational levels and filtered to simulate an average conductive hearing loss caused by OME. Results indicated significant differences in speech perception between filtered and unfiltered listening conditions in both quiet and noise. In fact, in noise the listeners with hearing loss consistent with OME obtained speech-perception scores of only 54%.

Recurrent OME in children has been linked to compromised speech, language, intellectual, attentional, learning, psychoeducational, and psychosocial development. Moreover, a relationship between recurrent OME and reductions in speech-perception ability has been reported. Gravel and Wallace (1992), for instance, examined the sentence recognition in noise (Pediatric Speech Intelligibility [PSI] Test) of four-year-old children with positive and negative histories of OME. Speech recognition was assessed with an adaptive procedure with the level of the sentences held constant at 60 dB SPL. Overall, the OME-positive children exhibited considerably greater difficulties understanding speech in a noisy environment than did the OME-negative group. Specifically, children with a positive history of OME required a significantly greater S/N ratio (2.9 dB) than did the OME-negative children to reach equivalent performance levels. Interestingly, a 2.9 dB decrease in sentence perception equates to a difference of approximately 24–29%.

CHILDREN WITH ARTICULATION DISORDERS

The most common communication disorder in childhood is errors in speech-sound production. Specifically, approximately 5–10% of all school-age children exhibit some difficulty in their oral production of speech. Children with articulation difficulties tend to demonstrate poorer speech perception in noise than do children with normal articulatory abilities (Crandell, McQuain, & Bess, 1987; Elliott, 1982). Unfortunately, there remains limited data on this subgroup of children with normal hearing. Elliott compared the speech-perception performance of children with articulation disorders to children with normal articulatory abilities. The SPIN high- and low-predictability sentence lists were presented binaurally to each child at several S/N ratios (+10, +5, and 0 dB). Although both groups of children obtained essentially 100% sentence-recognition scores in quiet, the performance of the children with articulation disorders was significantly poorer than in the normal control group. In fact, at an S/N ratio of +5 dB, which is commonly reported in classrooms, children with articulation disorders correctly recognized less than 50% of all sentence material presented (across all sentences presented), while the normal control group obtained sentence-recognition scores of approximately 65%.

CHILDREN WITH LANGUAGE DISORDERS, CHILDREN WITH AUDITORY PROCESSING DISORDERS, CHILDREN WITH LEARNING DISABILITIES, AND CHILDREN WITH ATTENTIONAL DISORDERS

Speech perception is dependent not only on receipt of specific acoustic information but also on the ability to relate these often ambiguous cues within the context of a language structure and use of circumstance. The cognitive activities that tie the acoustic signal to language are referred to as learning strategies by McCormick and Schiefelbusch (1984) and include selective attention, concept formation, and storage and retrieval, as discussed in Chapter 3. Breakdowns in the processes underlying the cognitive activities will impair the tie between the acoustic signal and language and so produce faulty perception.

Children with learning disabilities, language disorders, and auditory/attentional processing problems all have learning strategies that impair to one degree or another their ability to perceive or use acoustic signals in the classroom. The specific genesis of the problems for each learning strategy dysfunction is well beyond the scope of this chapter. There is, however, one commonality that might be susceptible to improvement through the use of sound field amplification.

Children who are learning disabled and language disordered and who have auditory processing and attention deficit problems frequently display an inability to attend to a desired acoustic signal. Often the inattention is derived from the fact that the desired signal is masked to some degree by surrounding ambient noise, or aspects of the signal simply are not loud enough to reach audibility. Amplifying the acoustic signal to improve the S/N ratio or to provide a completely audible acoustic spectrum might well serve to enable the child to focus on the relevant signal in the classroom and learn to ignore less intense, less relevant acoustic information. Unfortunately, there remains a lack of information regarding the effectiveness of sound field amplification on these populations of children.

CHILDREN WITH UNILATERAL SENSORINEURAL HEARING LOSS

Estimates suggest that approximately two to three of every one thousand children exhibit some degree of unilateral SNHL (Bess & Tharpe, 1986; Bess, Tharpe, & Gibler, 1986). Approximately 24–35% of these children have failed at least one grade in school. More than 13% require special education assistance. The educational difficulties experienced by these children may be explained, in part, by the perceptual difficulties they experience in the classroom. Specifically, children with unilateral SNHL often experience (1) speech-perception difficulties in noise and reverberation, particularly when speech is presented to the bad ear, and (2) an inability to localize a sound source.

Bess, Tharpe, and Gibler (1986), for example, examined speech perception in twenty-five children with mild to severe degrees of unilateral SNHL. Speech perception was assessed with consonant-vowel (CV) or vowel-consonant (VC) syllables from the Nonsense Syllable Test (NST) in several S/N ratios (quiet, +20, +10, 0, and −10 dB). The speech stimuli were presented to the children in frequently experienced classroom listening conditions: (1) monaural direct (speech directed at the good ear, noise presented to the bad ear), and (2) monaural indirect (noise presented to the good ear, speech presented to the good ear). While the children with unilateral hearing impairment performed similarly to the normal hearers in quiet, significant differences in perceptual ability were noted between the groups in the noisy listening conditions, particularly in the monaural indirect condition.

ACOUSTICAL STANDARDS FOR CHILDREN WITH NORMAL HEARING

Acoustical criteria for appropriate noise levels and reverberation times have not been well established for the diverse populations of normal-hearing children discussed above. Until additional research is conducted, a conservative standard for noise levels and reverberation times in listening environments for normal-hearing children should follow the same acoustical recommendations utilized for hearing-impaired listeners; that is, S/N ratios should surpass +15 dB and RTS should not exceed 0.4 second. The new ANSI standard for classroom acoustics is discussed in Chapter 7.

SUMMARY

This chapter has demonstrated that noise and reverberation levels characteristic of many classroom environments can cause significant reductions in the speech perception of not only children with hearing impairment but also children with normal hearing. If the accurate perception of speech is an important educational variable in pediatric listeners, then it is imperative that appropriate intervention strategies, such as sound field amplification, be incorporated into the classroom to assist these populations. This intervention will be discussed in the next chapter.

DISCUSSION TOPICS

1. Identify populations of children with normal hearing who experience speech-perception difficulties in the classroom. Discuss possible auditory and cognitive/linguistic hypotheses to explain why these perceptual difficulties are occurring.
2. Discuss habilitative procedures to improve speech perception for these populations in the classroom setting.
3. What acoustic criteria in terms of background noise level and reverberation time might you suggest for normal-hearing children who are at risk for listening and learning problems?
4. Do you think the currently accepted acoustic criteria for background noise and reverberation are appropriate? What changes would you make?

REFERENCES

Bergman, M. (1980). *Aging and the perception of speech.* Baltimore: University Park Press.

Bess, F. (1985). The minimally hearing-impaired child. *Ear and Hearing, 6,* 43–47.

Bess, F., Dodd-Murphy, J., & Parker, R. (1998). Children with minimal hearing loss: Prevalence, educational performance, and functional status. *Ear and Hearing, 19*(5), 339–354.

Bess, F., & McConnell, F. (1981). *Audiology, education and the hearing-impaired child.* St. Louis: C. V. Mosby.

Bess, F. H., & Tharpe, A. M. (1986). An introduction to unilateral sensorineural hearing loss in children. *Ear and Hearing, 7*(1), 3–13.

Bess, F. H., Tharpe, A. M., & Gibler, A. (1986). Auditory performance of children with unilateral sensorineural hearing loss. *Ear and Hearing, 7*(1), 20–26.

Boney, S., & Bess F. (1984). Noise and reverberation effects in minimal bilateral sensorineural hearing loss. Paper presented at the American Speech-Language-Hearing Association Convention, San Francisco, CA.

Crandell, C. (1991). Classroom acoustics for normal-hearing children: Implications for rehabilitation. *Educational Audiology Monograph, 2*(1), 18–38.

Crandell, C. (1992). Classroom acoustics for hearing-impaired children. *Journal of the Acoustical Society of America, 92*(4), 2470.

Crandell, C. (1993a). Speech recognition in noise by children with minimal hearing loss. *Ear and Hearing, 14*(3), 210–216.

Crandell, C. (1993b). A comparison of commercially available frequency modulation sound field amplification systems. *Educational Audiology Monograph, 3,* 15–30.

Crandell, C. (1996). The effects of sound field amplification on non-native English children. Submitted to *Educational Audiology Monograph, 4,* 1–5.

Crandell, C., & Bess, F. (1986). Speech recognition of children in a "typical" classroom setting. *American Speech, Language, & Hearing Association, 29,* 87.

Crandell, C., & Bess, F. (1987). Sound-field amplification in the classroom setting. *American Speech, Language, & Hearing Association, 29,* 87.

Crandell, C., & Flannagan, R. (1999). The effects of otitis media with effusion on speech perception in quiet and noise. *Journal of Educational Audiology, 6,* 28–32.

Crandell, C., McQuain, J., & Bess, F. (1987). Speech recognition of articulation-disordered children in noise and reverberation. Paper presented at the American Speech-Language-Hearing Association annual meeting, New Orleans, LA.

Crandell, C., & Smaldino, J. (1995a). The importance of room acoustics. In R. Tyler and D. Schum (Eds.), *Assistive listening devices* (pp. 142–164). Baltimore: Allyn and Bacon.

Crandell, C., & Smaldino, J. (1995b). An update of classroom acoustics for children with hearing impairment. *Volta Review, 6,* 18–25.

Crandell, C., Smaldino, J., & Flexer, C. (1995). *Sound field amplification: Theory and practical application.* Clifton Park, NY: Thomson Delmar Learning.

Davis, J., Elfenbein, J., Schum, R., & Bentler R. (1986). Effects of mild and moderate hearing impairments on language, educational, and psychosocial behavior of children. *Journal of Speech and Hearing Disorders, 51,* 53–62.

Dobie, R., & Berlin, C. (1979). Influence of otitis media on hearing and development. *Annuals of Otology, Rhinology, and Laryngology, 88,* 48–53.

Elliott, L. (1979). Performance of children aged 9 to 17 years on a test of speech intelligibility in noise using sentence material with controlled word predictability. *Journal of the Acoustical Society of America, 66,* 651–653.

Elliott, L. (1982). Effects of noise on perception of speech by children and certain handicapped individuals. *Sound and Vibration,* December, 9–14.

Elliott, L., Connors, S., Kille, E., Levin, S., Ball, K., & Katz, D. (1979). Children's understanding of monosyllabic nouns in quiet and in noise. *Journal of the Acoustical Society of America, 66,* 12–21.

Finitzo-Hieber, T. (1988). Classroom acoustics. In R. Roeser (Ed.), *Auditory disorders in school children* (2nd ed., pp. 221–233). New York: Thieme-Stratton.

Finitzo-Hieber, T., & Tillman, T. (1978). Room acoustics effects on monosyllabic word discrimination ability for normal and hearing-impaired children. *Journal of Speech and Hearing Research, 21,* 440–458.

Flexer, C., Millin, J., & Brown, L. (1990). Children with developmental disabilities: The effects of sound field amplification in word identification. *Language, Speech, and Hearing Services in the Schools, 21,* 177–182.

Gravel, J., & Wallace, I. (1992). Listening and language at 4 years of age: Effects of early otitis media. *Journal of Speech and Hearing Research, 35,* 220–228.

Johnson, C. E., Stein, R. L., Broadway, A., & Markwalter, T. S. (1996). "Minimal" high-frequency hearing loss and school-age children: Speech recognition in a classroom. *Language, Speech, and Hearing Services in the Schools, 28,* 77–85.

Leavitt, R. J., & Flexer, C. (1991). Speech degradation as measured by the rapid speech transmission index (RASTI). *Ear and Hearing, 12,* 115–118.

McCormick, L., & Schiefelbusch, R. (1984). *Early language intervention.* Columbus, OH: Merill Publishing.

Nabelek, A., & Nabelek, I. (1985). Room acoustics and speech perception. In J. Katz (Ed.), *Handbook of clinical audiology* (3rd ed.). Baltimore: Williams & Wilkins.

Nelson, E. C., Wasson, J. H., Johnson, D., & Hays, R. (1996). Dartmouth COOP functional health assessment charts: Brief measures for clinical practice. In B. Spilker (Ed.), *Quality of life and pharmacoeconomics in clinical trials* (2nd ed., pp. 161–168). Philadelphia: Lippencott-Raven Publishers.

Olsen, W. (1981). The effects of noise and reverberation on speech intelligibility. In F. H. Bess, B. A. Freeman, and J. S. Sinclair (Eds.), *Amplification in education.* Washington, DC: Alexander Graham Bell Association for the Deaf.

Olsen, W. (1988). Classroom acoustics for hearing-impaired children. In F. H. Bess (Ed.), *Hearing impairment in children.* Parkton, MD: York Press.

Ross, M. (1978). Classroom acoustics and speech intelligibility. In J. Katz (Ed.), *Handbook of clinical audiology.* Baltimore: Williams and Wilkins.

CHAPTER 5

Sound Field Amplification: A Comprehensive Literature Review

Gail Gegg Rosenberg, MS

KEY POINTS

- Sound field amplification is supported by efficacy studies that have demonstrated positive changes in students' literacy growth and academic achievement, speech-recognition abilities, attending skills, and learning behaviors.
- Benefits for the classroom teacher have been documented, as there were positive changes for the students as well as a decrease in vocal fatigue and vocal strain in teachers.
- Use of sound field amplification in the classroom has proven to be cost-effective.
- Positive outcomes that have resulted from use of sound field amplification include a reduction in special education referrals and fewer discipline incidents.
- Sound field amplification is often adopted as a prevention and intervention strategy based on the findings of efficacy studies.

Sound field amplification systems have been available in the marketplace for nearly thirty years. Slightly more than twenty years ago, definitive efficacy studies began to emerge, and over the past two decades more than fifty studies have been reported in the literature. In addition, it is not uncommon to read sound field success stories that are frequently reported in mainstream educational, technology, and other consumer print and electronic media.

Over the past five years, manufacturers have become very competitive in their offering of a variety of wireless and wired sound field infrared, FM, and VHF amplification devices. New options in loudspeaker and microphone technologies, signal processing, and signal transmission are emerging to meet the demands of audiologists, school districts, preschools, postsecondary institutions, and some public venue applications where there is a need to provide listeners with enhanced access to acoustic signals. Many of these forward-thinking applications of sound field technology have been the result of efficacy studies and have come about in response to product design requests by audiologists, other decision makers, and consumers.

This chapter contains a review of relevant research that chronicles the history of sound field amplification efficacy studies and also demonstrates the validity of this listening enhancement technology. Some researchers have concentrated on special populations, and others have sought to evaluate the effectiveness of sound field amplification in regular education classrooms. The efficacy of sound field amplification is supported by results of research studies that have demonstrated changes in students' literacy growth and academic achievement, speech-recognition abilities, attending skills, and learning behaviors. In addition, benefits for the classroom teacher have been well documented, as has the cost-effectiveness related to using this technology in the classroom. Other positive outcomes such as a reduction in special education referrals and fewer discipline incidents have been reported. Topics of national interest and attention, such as literacy, phonemic awareness, universal design, the No Child Left Behind efforts, the National Adult Literacy Survey (Kirsch, Jungeblut, Jenkins, & Kolstad, 1993), and the National Assessment Governing Board (NAGB) tend to invite the use of sound field amplification as a prevention and intervention strategy based on the findings of efficacy studies (Bourque & Byrd, 2000).

Although improvements in sound field technology have been documented over the past two decades, there has been a lack of empirical data available on the clinical practices of audiologists who recommend, dispense, install, and measure the efficacy of sound field technologies. Crandell and Smaldino (2000) reported data from 241 audiologists who completed a twenty-item questionnaire on current practices related to FM sound field technology. Respondents were primarily educational audiologists (82%), and 73% indicated that they only recommend sound field technologies. Table 5-1 summarizes other key survey findings related to decision-making practices, number and style of speakers preferred, provision of teacher in-service training, and the use of efficacy measures. Interestingly, the respondents revealed that commercially available efficacy tools were used only 25% of the time with teachers.

In addition to commercially available efficacy measures such as the Screening Instrument for Targeting Educational Risk (SIFTER) (Anderson, 1989) and the Listening Inventory for Education (LIFE) (Anderson &

TABLE 5-1 Summary of current practices in classroom sound field FM amplification by audiologists (N = 241) (Crandell & Smaldino, 2000)

Activity	Frequency
Recommend sound field technology	Recommend only: 73% Dispense and recommend: 19% Number of systems recommended per month: 2.4
Recommendations, observations, and training by audiologist	Recommends location: 83% Recommends number of speakers: 79% Installs system: 65% Considers Q factor in recommending speaker placement: 14% Observes classroom prior to placement: 72% Provides teacher in-service training: 87% Recommends acoustical modifications prior to placement: 32%
Number of speakers recommended	Four-speaker system: 39% Ceiling speaker: 14% Two- or three-speaker system: 9% Desktop: 7% One-speaker system: 5% Other arrangements such as distribution speakers: 17%
Microphone style	Boom microphone: 56% Lapel microphone: 21% Collar microphone: 18%
Teacher, parent, and student perception of sound field benefit	Speak to the teacher, parent, or student: 58%–62% Provide an efficacy measurement: 25% or less
Populations for which sound field amplification is recommended (40% and higher recommendation rate)	Conductive hearing loss: 69% Auditory processing disorder: 68% Minimal SNHL: 66% Younger children (< 13–15 years old): 63% Unilateral SNHL: 56% Mild SNHL: 52% Cochlear implant: 47% Attention deficit: 41%

Smaldino, 1998), researchers have used a variety of devised tools. The Listening and Learning Observation (LLO) was developed for the Improving Classroom Acoustics Project and has been used in other studies to gain information about teacher perceptions of students' listening behaviors, academic/preacademic skills, and academic/preacademic behaviors (DiSarno, Schowalter, & Grassa, 2002; Rosenberg et al., 1999). Surveys have also been devised to gain perceptions from teachers, students, parents, and administrators on the benefits of sound field amplification (Baldwin & Dougherty, 1997; Valente, 1998; Rosenberg et al., 1999). Other investigators have documented improvement based on a variety of efficacy measurement strategies and data collection methods, such as pre- and postperformance scores for a variety of speech-perception tests and academic growth demonstrated on national achievement tests and other standardized tests. The effects of distance from the speaker, various types of competing noise, and signal-to-noise (S/N) ratios mediated by sound field amplification have also been studied. Even though the body of sound field research continues to grow, audiologists and their colleagues need to continue to contribute to the knowledge base for the efficacious use of sound field technology as a prevention and intervention strategy.

SOUND FIELD AMPLIFICATION SYSTEM OPTIONS

The increase in options available for sound field amplification systems over the past five years has been discussed earlier in this book. The introduction of infrared sound field technology has led to comparisons with traditional FM sound field as well as innovations such as the bending wave speakers, digital signal processing, and the personal sound field systems. Several researchers have conducted studies on commercially available sound field amplification systems (Crandell, 1993; Mills, 1991; Prendergast, 2001).

Mills (1991) compared three systems (OMNI 2001 Wireless Classroom Amplification System, Lifeline Freefield Classroom Amplification System, and Phonic Ear Easy Listener Free Field Sound System) that were used for a two-month period with at-risk preschool and developmental kindergarten students. Teacher appraisal was used to determine which system was the most cost-effective and maintenance-free while providing high sound fidelity. None of the three systems was without some type of problem; however, the Phonic Ear Easy Listener Free Field system proved to be the most trouble-free and was easiest to operate and moderately priced.

Crandell (1993) focused on comparison of speech-recognition abilities of twenty children with normal hearing when using four available FM systems (Comtek OMNI 2001, Lifeline Freefield Classroom Amplification System,

Phonic Ear Easy Listener Free Field System, and Radio Shack). A three-speaker paradigm was used in a typical acoustical classroom environment. Acoustical analyses revealed relatively comparable frequency responses among the four systems. Speech-recognition results showed that while each system improved perception scores, there were differences among the systems. Specifically, the Radio Shack and Lifeline systems produced significantly higher speech-recognition scores than did either of the other two sound field FM amplification systems.

Prendergast (2001) conducted a study using the LightSPEED 500C traditional sound field system and compared student performance when using a single HI-Q loudspeaker and the HI-Q bending wave single loudspeaker. Results of the study demonstrated significant differences in high-frequency energy preservation in a classroom setting in addition to differences in speech discrimination performance by third- and fourth-grade students when using the bending wave speaker. An informal assessment of the students' speaker preference indicated that they felt the performance of the bending wave speaker was superior.

Crandell, Charlton, Kinder, and Kriesman (2001) compared listening in noise capabilities of twenty young adults under unaided and aided listening conditions and found that the Phonic Ear Easy Listener body-worn personal FM system produced higher scores than the Phonic Ear Toteable sound field system that was placed on a desk.

LITERACY AND ACADEMIC ACHIEVEMENT STUDIES

Efficacy studies on the positive effects of sound field amplification on growth in literacy and academic achievement have been conducted on listeners with normal hearing and those with hearing loss. Participants in these studies ranged from preschool age for the early-literacy experiment to students in college-level audiology and aural rehabilitation courses. According to Levitt and Ross (2002), sound field systems are, at least in part, responsible for removing some of the strain from the auditory learning process. Table 5-2 summarizes these studies.

The original investigation on sound field amplification was the three-year longitudinal project called Mainstream Amplification Resource Room Study (MARRS), conducted in the Wabash and Ohio Valley schools in southern Illinois between 1977 and 1980 (Sarff, 1981). The MARRS project compared academic progress of students in grades four through six who received treatment under different amplification conditions. These groups of students were examined for (1) minimal to mild hearing loss (pure-tone thresholds between 10 and 40 dB HL), (2) coexisting learning deficit, and (3) normal learning potential. Approximately half of the children remained in regular classrooms

TABLE 5-2 Summary of sound field efficacy studies demonstrating student improvement in literacy and academic achievement

Investigators	Student Population	Improvement in Academic Achievement Obtained with Sound Field Amplification
Sarff (1981); Ray, Sarff, & Glassford (1984)	MARRS project (fourth- through sixth-grade students with minimal hearing loss, academic deficit, and normal learning potential)	The MARRS project demonstrated that students with minimal hearing loss and learning disabilities in amplified classrooms made significant academic gains at a faster rate, to a higher level, and at one-tenth the cost of students in unamplified classrooms and receiving traditional pull-out resource-room intervention.
Ray (1992)	MARRS validation (fourth through sixth graders with minimal hearing loss and academic deficit)	Students with minimal hearing loss instructed in unamplified classrooms performed academically at an average 0.4 SD below normal. Students with minimal hearing loss in amplified classrooms performed at or above average.
Flexer (1989, 1992); Osborn, VonderEmbse, & Graves (1989)	MARCS project (kindergarten through third graders in regular education classes)	Students in classes with FM sound field amplification achieved higher scores in listening, vocabulary, math concepts, and math computation on the Iowa Test of Basic Skills, with greater gains made by younger students.
Schermer (1991)	First-grade students with normal hearing and minimal hearing loss	Higher reading test scores were attained by students with minimal to mild hearing loss in amplified classrooms, and decreased posttest scores were identified for students with known minimal to mild hearing loss in unamplified classrooms.
Howell (1996)	Fifteen normal-hearing, regular education third graders	Significant improvement was noted in test scores when teacher used sound field FM to present new information.

(continued)

TABLE 5-2 *(continued)*

Investigators	Student Population	Improvement in Academic Achievement Obtained with Sound field Amplification
Valente (1998)	Sixty-four college students enrolled in audiology and aural rehabilitation classes	Use of sound field amplification showed significant differences among test scores for the audiology course at the fourth exam and the final exam, with similar results for the aural rehabilitation course.
Anderson (1999)	Two case studies of students with severe to profound hearing loss	Indicators suggest that early-grade performance cannot be used to predict performance in later grades, progress must be systematically monitored, and caution should be exercised in the use of sound field amplification over other hearing assistive technologies.
Darai (2000)	First-grade students (eighty-five experimental, eighty-one control) in eight regular education classrooms	Students in amplified classrooms achieved greater literacy gains than control students, particularly bilingual and special education students, on the Informal Reading Inventory. Teachers noted positive change on the LIFE due to FM sound field intervention.
Long and Flexer (2001)	Thirty-seven kindergarten through fifth-grade regular education classrooms	Referral rates for special education decreased from 7.72% to 4.6% after thirty-seven classrooms were amplified with sound field technology.
Flexer, Biley, Hinkley, Harkema, & Holcomb (2002)	Fifty-three students in three prekindergarten and three kindergarten classes	Results revealed a trend toward enhanced development of phonemic awareness skills when phonemic awareness instruction was augmented with sound field amplification. The least number of at-risk readers were found in the amplified preschool and kindergarten classrooms.

(continued)

TABLE 5-2 *(continued)*

Investigators	Student Population	Improvement in Academic Achievement Obtained with Sound field Amplification
McCarty & Gertel (2003)	Fifth-grade high-need students in regular classes	SAT scores improved +12% to +20% for reading, math, language, science, and social studies with a +14% improvement in total test battery in the first year, followed in second year by an average 10% improvement over first-year results.
Loven, Fisk, & Johnson (2003)	Forty-eight students in two regular education second-grade classes	Three appraisals of academic achievement over a six-month period showed significantly better performance on reading and spelling for students in the amplified classroom but no significant differences for mathematics.

where sound field FM amplification systems were in use; the remaining children received traditional instruction in unamplified rooms. The two-speaker sound field FM system was used an average of three hours per day. Both groups showed gains in reading, language arts, and total composite scores based on Scientific Research Associates (SRA) Achievement Series test data. However, the greatest improvement was documented for the group instructed in amplified classrooms. Not only did these students show significant gains in academic achievement, but they also were noted to achieve in reading and language arts at a faster rate, to a higher level, and at one-tenth the cost of students taken from regular classes and provided instruction in a resource-room setting. Also important is that the younger students (fourth and fifth graders) showed the greatest degree of academic growth. The MARRS project achieved national validation status in 1981 as part of the National Diffusion Network of the U.S. Department of Education and was recertified in 1992 (Ray, 1987; Ray, Sarff, & Glassford, 1984; Sarff, 1981).

Following the landmark MARRS study, the use of FM sound field amplification was introduced as an innovative prevention and intervention strategy in classrooms for students with normal hearing as well as students judged to be at risk for listening and learning problems. Project MARRS continues to function as part of the National Diffusion Network and offers assistance to adoption sites. Adoption data validated in 1992 supported previous findings that students with minimal hearing loss who are instructed in unamplified classrooms perform academically at an average level approximately 0.4 standard deviations (SD) below normal. Students with minimal hearing loss in amplified classrooms were found to perform at or above average (Ray, 1992).

Over a three-year period, the Putnam County Ohio Office of Education investigated the efficiency and cost-effectiveness of sound field amplification for improving the quality and consistency of oral instruction for lower-grade elementary children in nine rural school districts in Ohio (Flexer, 1989, 1992; Osborn, VonderEmbse, & Graves, 1989). Project MARCS (Mainstream Amplification Regular Classroom Study) utilized the OMNI 2001 sound field FM amplification system with a two-speaker paradigm in seventeen kindergarten through third-grade classrooms matched with seventeen unamplified classrooms. Results of the Iowa Test of Basic Skills (TBS) indicated higher achievement levels for students in the experimental classrooms in the following subtest areas by grade level for the first year: listening and language (kindergarten and first grade), vocabulary (first grade), math concepts (second and third grades), and math computation (third grade). For the second year, significant findings were reported for experimental classrooms in three of the four grades: word analysis (kindergarten and first grade), math concepts (first and third grades), math problem-solving (first grade), and math computation (third grade). A general trend showed that the younger the student, the greater the difference between the achievement test scores of the control group and the experimental group. Those students who failed to pass puretone and tympanometry screening and were placed in unamplified classes showed the poorest overall performance on the TBS.

Classroom observations were also a part of Project MARCS. Experimental findings indicated that the use of sound field FM amplification encouraged teacher mobility, increased the number of students participating, produced a more consistent teacher rate of speech, and showed better student transition between classroom activities and general activity levels. There were fewer special education referrals and learning disabilities placements in the schools with the greatest number of sound field FM amplification systems in the lower elementary grades. Informal MARCS evaluation by teachers in experimental classrooms generally indicated more consistent student attending skills, a reduction in teacher vocal strain and voice fatigue, and increased versatility in instructional techniques. At the end of three years, forty-six classrooms were using sound field FM amplification, which suggests that these educators were convinced that it was helping students listen and learn better.

Schermer (1991) conducted a study of reading achievement in first-grade students. Results showed higher achievement on the Gates-MacGinitie Reading Tests for students in amplified classrooms, particularly for students with primarily mild, fluctuating conductive hearing losses. Students with known mild hearing loss who were not placed in amplified classrooms showed a decrease on posttest scores. A recommendation of this study was to explore the effectiveness of sound field FM amplification as an alternative to special education personnel required for resource-room instruction. We now know that sound field FM amplification is a viable alternative that will meet placement requirements for many students with known hearing loss. Subsequently, this allows other students in the class to benefit from the enhanced access to auditory information.

Undergraduate students (N = 64) used sound field amplification in audiology and aural rehabilitation courses during a portion of each course in a study reported by Valente (1998). The Phonic Ear Easy Listener four-speaker sound field system was used with the instructor wearing a directional lapel microphone. A 7 dB SPL enhancement was produced to amplify the instructor's voice during lectures. The study compared mean examination scores under amplified and unamplified conditions. For the audiology course, improvement was seen with exam 4 and in the aural rehabilitation course with exam 2 following the implementation of the sound field system. Students and instructors completed a ten-item questionnaire for each of the four semesters that the sound field amplification was in use. Mean responses from the questionnaires showed a positive, or at least a neutral, tendency. Subjective student comments included greater attentiveness, decreased distractibility, less reliance on selective seating in order to hear clearly, and clearer reception of the instructor's voice. Subjective comments from the instructor corroborated the students' opinion that they were more attentive and interactive, and the instructor also noted a decrease in vocal strain when using the sound field amplification.

Anderson (1999) reported two case studies of mainstreamed students with hearing loss who used sound field amplification over a period of several years. One student had a severe-to-profound bilateral hearing loss, and the other presented with a moderate-to-severe mixed hearing loss bilaterally. Both students were assessed as being capable of at least average school performance with some aural rehabilitation support. Both students rejected the use of personal FM systems, and each used at least one working hearing aid. Word discrimination in noise was assessed as being fair to good when augmented with visual clues. In the fourth grade, the students were introduced to a wireless FM; one student showed appreciable gains, while the other rejected it after a few weeks. The students were periodically monitored using the SIFTER and LIFE protocols. While a two-subject study is limited in its ability to provide definitive data on the use of sound field versus personal FM systems for children with moderate or greater levels of hearing loss, there are some good points to be made: (1) early-grade performance by children who are hard of hearing cannot be used to predict performance as they progress academically; (2) serial teacher-observation forms (e.g., SIFTER, LIFE) provide valuable information to support a change in amplification options; (3) the S/N ratio from the sound field system apparently was not adequate for the students to follow directions as academic demands increased; and (4) caution should be exercised in recommending sound field amplification as an alternative to other technologies for students with moderate or greater degrees of hearing loss.

Concern about classroom acoustics and the impact on reading, such as the need for a favorable S/N ratio in order to clearly hear the phonetic markers for identifying differences between words and learning the correct pronunciation of unknown words, were underlying issues in the study by Darai (2000). This investigator used sound field FM systems to demonstrate improvement in literacy scores of first-grade students. Participants in the study were 166 students (85 experimental, 81 control) in four experimental and four control first-grade classrooms in the Broward County, Florida, school district. The Phonic Ear Easy Listener four-speaker FM sound field system was installed in the four experimental classrooms for a five-month period. The Informal Reading Inventory (IRI) was used as the efficacy measure by comparing midyear and end-of-year instructional reading levels to demonstrate literacy growth. Results showed significantly greater literacy gains for students in the experimental classrooms, particularly for bilingual and special education students. A second efficacy tool, the Teacher Appraisal of Listening Difficulty Inventory of the Listening Inventory for Education (LIFE), was completed by the classroom teachers and overwhelmingly indicated positive changes in attention, classroom participation, and learning. In addition, teachers in the experimental classroom reported that the improved classroom acoustics provided by the sound field system enhanced instruction in both phonics and language.

Long and Flexer (2001) reported that special education referrals declined by nearly 50% after thirty-seven elementary classrooms (kindergarten through fifth grade) received sound field amplification and used the sound enhancement technology for an eight-month period. After using sound field amplification, the average special education referral rate of 4.6% was a significant decline from the average 7.72% referral rate for the nine previous academic years. As a result of these positive findings, the Onconto Falls, Wisconsin, school district has included sound field amplification in its universal design approach, which specifies that this technology can be implemented by general education teachers and not specifically special education teachers. Another positive outcome was that the district expanded its universal design plan to include sound enhancement amplification in all middle school classrooms.

An interesting study by Flexer et al. (2002) was designed to determine if early phonological and phonemic awareness training coupled with the use of sound field amplification would yield a reduction in the number of children identified as at-risk readers on the Yopp-Singer Test of Phonemic Segmentation (Yopp, 1995). Emphasis on immersion of preschool children in phonemic and phonological awareness is a common trend today to promote early literacy development. Three classes of typical four-year-olds participated in this year-long Ohio study where students were identified and tracked through the end of their first semester in kindergarten. Each group received different early phonological and phonemic awareness interventions. Group A (control group, N = 23) received the school district's standard preschool and kindergarten curriculum. Group B (phonological and phonemic awareness group, N = 7) received direct group phonological and phonemic awareness instruction four times weekly. Group C (phonological and phonemic awareness group, N = 23) received the same intervention as Group B and was provided with sound field amplification. Teachers in Groups B and C received in-service on phonological awareness, and teachers in Group C received additional in-service on sound field amplification. Four-speaker Audio Enhancement Ultimate infrared systems were installed in a Group C prekindergarten classroom and a kindergarten classroom. Results showed that both Groups B and C achieved significantly higher scores on the Yopp-Singer Test than students in Group A. Trends observed in this study suggest that (1) the sound field system produced a more consistent positive effect across Group C than the treatments used in Groups A and B, (2) the level of homogeneity in Group C established the students as being less at risk for reading problems than children in the other two groups, and (3) phonological and phonemic awareness training to promote early literacy development was more effective when sound field amplification was used.

The effects of sound field amplification on specific educational goals were reported by Massie (2003) on a study that involved 242 children in twelve second-grade classes in Australia. The children had no prior experience with sound field amplification, and 61% were of another family language background. Eight classrooms received sound field amplification alternating "on" and "off" with crossover at midyear, and the remaining four classes were amplified for the entire year, alternating between single and dual teacher microphones. Teachers received in-service training prior to the experiment. Results showed significant improvement in literacy (i.e., reading and writing) and math when sound field amplification was in use. Findings were greater when students were assessed after experiencing sound field in the "on" first/"off" last rather than the "off" first/"on" last test condition. This finding suggests that the timing of the sound field intervention is important.

Results of a two-year study reported by McCarty and Gertel (2003) clearly demonstrate a reverse trend in failing scores by fifth-grade high-need students on the Stanford Achievement Test (SAT). Sound field amplification was introduced to classrooms where students had shown declining scores on the SAT; however, following the implementation of the sound enhancement technology, SAT scores for fifth-grade students improved an average of 12% in reading, 14% in math, 17% in language, 20% in science and social studies with an overall test battery increase of 14%. Even greater gains of an average additional 10% increase were documented during the second year for students in the amplified classrooms. An additional finding showed that sound field amplification coupled with phonemic and phonological awareness training reduced the number of students identified as at-risk learners.

Significant improvement in reading and spelling by second-grade students in an amplified classroom were revealed in a study by Loven, Fisk, and Johnson (2003). Appraisals of student achievement in three core academic areas (reading, spelling, mathematics) were conducted three times during a six-month period for forty-eight students in two regular education second-grade classrooms—one amplified, the other unamplified—in Minnesota. While significant gains were shown by students in the amplified classroom for reading and spelling, t-tests did not show a difference between the classrooms for mathematics. These investigators also obtained two subjective measures of student listening behaviors, and a two-way ANOVA showed a significant interaction for the two main variables of room treatment and time. Comparison of pretreatment and during-treatment measures revealed findings similar to other studies in that students demonstrated a robust increase in attending behaviors following installation of the FM sound field amplification.

SPEECH-RECOGNITION STUDIES

There has been a proliferation of studies on the benefits of sound field amplification on the speech-recognition capabilities of a variety of subjects and under a range of conditions. This section discusses research that highlights the positive effects of sound field amplification on speech-recognition performance in the following categories: (1) distance from the speaker, (2) general education classrooms, (3) listeners with hearing loss, (4) listeners with cochlear implants, (5) other special needs populations, (6) young adults, and (7) innovative sound field technologies. Refer to Table 5-3 for a summary of studies demonstrating the effects of sound field amplification on speech recognition.

Speech Recognition and Distance

Crandell and Bess (1986) were the first to report findings of improved speech-recognition scores when students used sound field FM amplification. These authors examined its benefits for twenty students with normal hearing in a typical classroom setting (S/N ratio of +6 dB; reverberation time [RT] of 0.6 second at 6, 12, and 24 feet). Results showed significant improvement in students' ability to recognize sentence information under the amplified condition at 12 and 24 feet from a speaker.

TABLE 5-3   Summary of sound field efficacy studies demonstrating improvement in speech-recognition skills

Investigators	Student Population	Improvement in Speech Recognition Obtained with Sound Field Amplification
Crandell & Bess (1986)	Twenty students with normal hearing	Students showed significant improvement in sentence recognition ability under the amplified condition in typical classrooms (S/N = +6 dB, RT = 0.6 sec).
Blair, Myrup, & Viehweg (1989)	Ten students (CA = 7–14 yrs) with mild to moderate SNHL	Students with mild to moderate SNHL demonstrated an average of 12% improvement in word-recognition score when using personal hearing aids with FM sound field over hearing aids alone.
Jones, Berg, & Viehweg (1989)	Kindergarten students with normal hearing (N = 18) and mild hearing loss (N = 18)	Use of FM sound field amplification decreased student-teacher distance and produced word-recognition scores comparable to close listening at 4 feet.
Flexer, Millin, & Brown (1990)	Primary school-age children with developmental disabilities	Developmentally disabled students with history of persistent conductive hearing loss exhibited improved word-recognition scores.
Neuss, Blair, & Viehweg (1991)	Students with minimal hearing loss	Students with minimal hearing loss showed improved word-recognition scores in noise when using sound field amplification vs. personal hearing aids.
Crandell (1993)	Twenty students with normal hearing	Significantly higher word-recognition scores were achieved by students at distances of 12 and 24 feet when using sound field amplification.
Zabel & Tabor (1993)	145 regular education third- through fifth-grade students	Students achieved improved spelling test scores under FM sound field amplification in quiet and under degraded listening at a +12 dB S/N ratio.

(continued)

TABLE 5-3 *(continued)*

Investigators	Student Population	Improvement in Speech Recognition Obtained with Sound Field Amplification
Crandell (1996)	Twenty nonnative English-speaking children	Improved speech-perception scores . were achieved at distances of 12 and 24 feet when using sound field amplification.
Poissant, Brackett, & Maxon (1998)	Twenty children (ten with normal hearing using mild-gain hearing aids, ten with multichannel cochlear implants)	FM sound field amplification partially restored acoustical cues obliterated by distance and noise, making it easier for cochlear implant users in the mainstream to accurately perceive speech.
Smaldino, Green, & Nelson (1997)	Thirty-one normal-hearing college students in a phonetics class	Significantly fewer fine auditory discrimination errors occurred with. sound field amplification at approximately +10 dB than in unamplified condition.
Crandell, Holmes, Flexer, & Payne (1998)	Eight children and ten adults with cochlear implants	Traditionally placed sound field system did not significantly augment speech recognition for listeners with cochlear implants on any of four subtests of the Early Speech Perception Test Battery under any of four listening conditions.
Allcock (1999)	Three amplified and two unamplified elementary classrooms in New Zealand	After eight weeks of sound field amplification use, students in amplified classrooms showed a 65–74% improvement of ≥ 1 stanine on the Test of Phonological Awareness compared to students in unamplified classes showing a 46% improvement of ≥ 1 stanine.
Gordon-Langbein & Metinger (1999)	Two elementary classrooms	Students' abilities to identify initial consonant phonemes in words, using recorded questions, improved by 45% in the amplified condition.

(continued)

TABLE 5-3 *(continued)*

Investigators	Student Population	Improvement in Speech Recognition Obtained with Sound Field Amplification
Eriks-Brophy & Ayukawa (2000)	Twenty second- and third-grade students (ten with hearing loss and ten age-matched peers)	Significant improvements in speech intelligibility were noted for recognition of Inuttitut syllables by both groups of students when using sound field amplification.
Lederman, Johnson, Crandell, & Smaldino (2000)	Seventy-two third-grade students (ELL, at-risk, special education) and nine third- through fifth-grade hard-of-hearing students	Significant improvement on sixteen of forty listening tasks (words and CV syllables) and conditions (S/N at –6, 0, +6 dB) using the SmartSpeaker "Intelligence" digital signal processing sound field system with ambient noise compensation (ANC) capability.
Crandell, Charlton, Kinder, & Kreisman (2001)	Twenty young adults (mean CA = 21.8) with normal hearing	The HINT test was presented in noise under unaided, portable sound field, and personal body-worn FM listening conditions. Speech-perception scores improved using both FM systems and were significantly better with the body-worn system.
Prendergast (2001)	Thirty-one third-grade and thirty-three fourth-grade students with normal hearing	Enhanced performance was shown by all children on the California Consonant Test using the bending wave speaker vs. a traditional sound field speaker.
Bennetts & Flynn (2002)	Four students with Down syndrome	Speech-perception performance improved significantly in all aided listening conditions.
Mendel, Roberts, & Walton (2003)	128 regular education kindergarten students with normal hearing	Two-year study showed significant and immediate improvement in speech perception and accelerated development of speech perception in noise by students in amplified classrooms.
Updike & Conner (2003)	495 first-grade students in regular education classes	Significant improvement in Goldman-Fristoe Test of Auditory Discrimination scores in quiet (76% to 92%) and noise (60% to 84%).

Performance of 145 normal-hearing third, fourth, and fifth graders on spelling tests under unamplified and amplified conditions was reported by Zabel and Tabor (1993). The unamplified listening condition was presented at 0 dB S/N ratio (typical classroom) and at +12 dB S/N ratio in the amplified condition. The Lifeline sound field system with a four-speaker arrangement was used during amplified testing. The investigators used tape-recorded Curriculum-Based Measurement spelling tests and found that all classes immediately achieved significant improvement in spelling scores under amplified conditions at close and distant seating, with improvement increasing with distance.

Crandell (1993) evaluated commercially available sound field FM amplification systems as a function of students' word-recognition scores at various speaker-listener distances of 6, 12, and 24 feet. Findings showed that compared to unamplified listening, speech-recognition scores were enhanced using each of the FM systems. In addition, students achieved elevated word-recognition scores in the amplified treatment at speaker-listener distances of 12 and 24 feet.

Speech Recognition in General Education Classrooms

Gordon-Langbein and Metinger (1999) reported on a study conducted in two classrooms at Rolling Hills Elementary School. The purpose of the study was to determine if sound field amplification would improve auditory discrimination skills in the classroom. The stimuli were two sets of tape-recorded questions designed to assess the children's ability to identify initial consonant phonemes in spoken words. Students were assessed in the unamplified and amplified conditions, and results showed an average 45% improvement in the amplified condition and an average 42% deficit under the unamplified condition.

A study funded by the Oticon Foundation was undertaken in two schools in New Zealand. Purposes of this study reported by Allcock (1999) related to the following benefits of sound field amplification: (1) improvement in S/N ratio in classrooms, (2) increase in on-task behavior for children with normal hearing and children with hearing loss, and (3) improved ability to discriminate between speech sounds in words. Based on data from three classrooms, an improvement of 5–10 dB in S/N ratio was documented. To examine on-task behavior, an eight-week observation was conducted with sound field amplification being alternately used for two-week segments (i.e., two weeks on, two weeks off). It was found that when the sound field amplification was in use, on-task behavior ranged from being 14% less on task to 50% more on task, with a mean of 18% more on-task time than when the system was off. Findings were similar for children with normal hearing and those with hearing loss. The final aspect of this study was to examine the children's ability to identify differences between speech sounds as measured by pre- and posttesting with the Test of Phonological Awareness. Students in amplified classrooms showed a 65–74% improvement of one stanine or more compared to students in unamplified classes who showed only an average 46% improvement of one stanine or more.

First-grade children (N = 495) participated in a study to measure the effectiveness of infrared sound field amplification on auditory discrimination abilities using the Goldman-Fristoe Test of Auditory Discrimination (Updike & Conner, 2003). Pre- and postclassroom amplification measures were taken under both quiet and white competing noise (+ 5 dB S/N) conditions. Significant improvement was found for both listening conditions, with an average improvement of 16% in quiet (72–88%) and 32% under the competing noise condition (48–80%). Data was further analyzed to show improvements for not only those students without disabilities (quiet, 72–88%; noise, 48–80%), but also for students with special needs (quiet, 72–84%; noise, 50–76%). For the noise condition, findings were significant for students diagnosed with learning disability, attention deficit disorder, hearing loss, and speech-language disorder. Under neither listening condition was a significant finding found for students identified with mental handicap, auditory processing disorder, or emotional disorder. A secondary purpose of this study was to provide data to local school administrators and grant-funding agencies about the benefits of sound field amplification on students' listening and auditory discrimination abilities.

A study reported by Mendel, Roberts, and Walton (2003) evaluated the effectiveness of the Easy Listener FM sound field system on speech perception in young children across treatment groups longitudinally. Participants were 128 kindergarten students with normal hearing in general education classrooms, with 95 students participating through the duration of the two-year study. Students were randomly assigned to the treatment group in three classrooms with sound field amplification, and the control group was comprised of three unamplified classrooms during the first year. Classrooms were initially selected on the basis of similarity of size, shape, and acoustic parameters. As the students moved into first grade, four classes were amplified and four served as controls. Students were monitored through the end of first grade. The Word Intelligibility Picture Identification Test (WIPI) presented in the presence of recorded noise from the classrooms was used to measure speech-perception performance. The only condition that produced a significant finding was the markedly better performance by the treatment group for the two assessments taken during kindergarten. By the end of first grade, there was no significant difference for group performance on the WIPI. For both groups, there was essentially no difference when stimuli were presented without the benefit of sound field amplification. The authors infer that improvement in speech perception appears to be affected more by the increased signal enhancement provided by sound field amplification than by its long-term use. When using the PBK test as stimuli, there was no significant difference between the groups across test sessions. By the end of the study, the control group did appear to bridge the gap in regard to speech-recognition abilities, thus reinforcing the immediate benefit of sound field amplification for the treatment group. These investigators caution that maturation did play a role in the measurable improvements for both groups but stressed that the immediate enhanced performance by students in the amplified classrooms could be attributed to the use of sound field amplification.

Speech Recognition by Students with Hearing Loss

Blair, Myrup, and Viehweg (1989) compared word-recognition abilities of ten students (ages seven through fourteen years) with mild-to-moderate sensorineural hearing loss under three conditions: (1) personal hearing aids in conjunction with a two-speaker sound field system, (2) personal hearing aids coupled via miniloop to a personal FM system, and (3) personal hearing aids only. These investigators used a two-speaker ceiling-mounted presentation to achieve sound field FM amplification. Use of personal hearing aids in conjunction with a sound field FM amplification system yielded an average improvement of 12% in word-recognition scores compared to those obtained when students used only personal hearing aids. However, the greatest gain in word-recognition scores was achieved when students used their hearing aids coupled with personal FM systems; this resulted in an additional 5% improvement over the sound field FM amplification condition. These findings clearly support use of a sound field FM amplification system as an additional tool for access to auditory information for students with properly functioning hearing aids. The investigation did not examine use of a personal FM system in conjunction with the sound field FM amplification system, which is a common practice in schools today.

The effects of speaker-listener distance and sound field FM amplification on the speech perception of eighteen normal-hearing and eighteen kindergarten students with mild sensorineural hearing loss were studied by Jones, Berg, and Viehweg (1989). Students were given a speech-recognition test under three conditions: (1) twelve feet from the tape player, (2) four feet from the tape player, and (3) sound field FM amplification via ceiling-mounted speakers. Results revealed significantly higher perception scores for both groups under the close (four feet) and sound field FM amplification listening conditions compared to distant listening at twelve feet. Although the average sound field score was slightly higher than the average close-listening score, significant differences were not seen. This study demonstrated the advantage of improving the S/N ratio in kindergarten classrooms either by physically decreasing the student-teacher distance or by using sound field FM amplification.

Neuss, Blair, and Viehweg (1991) investigated the word-recognition abilities of students with minimal hearing loss under three listening conditions:

(1) personal hearing aid only, (2) unaided, and (3) sound field FM amplification only. Students had pure-tone averages between 15 and 40 dB HL and were hearing aid users. A Realistic sound field FM amplification system with a three-speaker arrangement was used to provide amplification in this study. Monosyllabic word-recognition scores obtained in noise showed significant improvement when students used sound field FM amplification but not when personal hearing aids were used.

A pilot project to examine the benefits of sound field amplification for speech intelligibility and on-task behavior measures in classrooms of Inuit students of Nunavik, California, was undertaken by Eriks-Brophy and Ayu-kawa (2000). Concern about the incidence of otitis media (28% of the school-age population) inspired this pilot study. The Phonic Ear Easy Listener four-speaker sound field system was installed in three classrooms for a three-month period and set to achieve at least a +6 dB S/N ratio. This study compared the performance of students with normal hearing to age-matched students with hearing loss using observations of four categories of attending behaviors. For the speech intelligibility portion of the study, ten students with hearing loss were compared with age-matched peers on a recorded test of Inuttitut syllables, and both groups showed significant improvement in the amplified condition. On-task behavior was also assessed, and improvement was documented for six of seven students, with all students showing improvement in at least one attending behavior category. Overall, findings support the potential benefits of sound field amplification for multicultural populations who face communication access challenges related to hearing loss and learning a second language. Teachers also identified the following benefits from use of the sound field amplification: increased attention in large group lessons, increased student response time, increased student participation in class discussions, decreased need for repetition of information, improved listening behaviors, and decreased teacher fatigue at the end of the day.

Speech Recognition by Listeners with Cochlear Implants

Use of FM sound field amplification with children using cochlear implants found differing results. Some children experience difficulty using personal FM systems coupled with their cochlear implant. Poissant, Brackett, and Maxon (1998) explored the possibility of using a personal sound field FM system to accommodate listening difficulties imposed by distance from the speaker and environmental noise. The purposes of this study were to (1) document change in feature recognition in noise and (2) determine the amount of increased noise tolerance. Ten normal hearing children fit with mild-gain hearing aids and ten mainstreamed children with multichannel cochlear implants participated in the study. The researchers found that noise has a greater detrimental effect than distance on the phoneme perception ability of cochlear implant users. Isophonemic word lists were presented at 65 dB HL via monitored live voice. When using the Omni Petite personal FM system placed on the child's desk, both groups achieved a similar degree of improvement in phoneme perception scores. Children with normal hearing improved from 73% to 93%, and children with cochlear implants improved from 44% to 65%. As noise levels increased, both groups experienced an equivalent amount of degradation in phoneme perception. Results of this study indicate that for children with cochlear implants, a personal FM sound field system partially restores acoustic cues that are distorted by the effects of distance and noise, which is a positive accommodation in the mainstream education setting.

The Crandell, Holmes, Flexer, and Payne (1998) study sought to investigate the effects of a traditionally placed FM sound field amplification system on the speech-recognition abilities of eight children and ten adult listeners with cochlear implants. Material from the Early Speech Perception Test Battery (ESPT) (Moog & Geers, 1990; Nilsson, Soli, & Sullivan, 1994) was used to evaluate speech-recognition performance. Testing was conducted in a typical classroom acoustical environment under four listening conditions: (1) quiet, (2) quiet with FM sound field amplification, (3) noise, and (4) noise with FM sound field amplification. The ESPT speech stimuli were delivered via monitored live voice at approximately 83 dB SPL. Multitalker babble was introduced to the classroom environment for the two competing noise conditions at a +6 dB S/N. The Audio Enhancement Omni Deluxe FM sound field system was used with a four-speaker arrangement. Findings of this study demonstrated that the traditionally placed FM sound field amplification did not significantly augment speech recognition for either the pediatric or adult listeners across the four experimental listening conditions. The investigators suggested that additional noise reduction strategies be explored to improve speech-recognition abilities of cochlear implant users under noise and quiet listening conditions.

Speech Recognition by Other Special Needs Populations

Flexer, Millin, and Brown (1990) examined the effects of sound field FM amplification on word identification by primary-age children with developmental disabilities. An SRT-100 Classroom Acoustic Sound Field System was used with a two-speaker design. Audiological evaluation data indicated that only one of the nine students had normal hearing sensitivity or normal immittance results. Six students had histories of persistent hearing loss and had been referred repeatedly for medical treatment. Results indicated that these youngsters with developmental disabilities achieved significant improvement in word-recognition scores under the amplified listening condition. In the unamplified condition, students made nearly three times as many errors as in the amplified listening condition.

Greater speech-perception difficulties are experienced by children for whom English is a second language (ESL) than by native English-speaking children (Crandell and Smaldino, 1996). In a study by Crandell (1996), the effects of FM sound field amplification on the perceptual abilities of ESL children (native Spanish speakers) in a typical acoustical classroom environment were examined. Participants were twenty nonnative English-speaking children whose monosyllabic word perception was evaluated at three speaker-listener distances. The classroom S/N ratio was +6 dB with a reverberation time (RT) of 0.6 seconds. Recorded Phonetically Balanced Kindergarten (PBK-50s) monosyllabic words were the test stimuli, and a twelve-speaker multitalker babble was used as the competing noise. The students were tested under unamplified and amplified conditions at distances of six, twelve, and twenty-four feet. During the amplified condition, a Lifeline Free Field Amplification System calibrated to achieve a 10 dB increase in sound pressure level was used with a four-speaker arrangement. Results showed that the ESL children demonstrated more speech-perception difficulties in the unamplified listening condition, especially at distances of twelve and twenty-four feet, which is comparable to being seated in the middle to rear portion of the classroom. For the amplified condition, speech-perception scores were significantly enhanced, improving from 64.7% to 80.6% at a distance of twelve feet and from 49.2% to 79.1% at a distance of twenty-four feet. In the amplified condition, the children's speech-perception scores remained essentially constant across each speaker-to-listener distance.

The efficacy of sound field amplification to provide improved access to the speech signal for children with Down syndrome was investigated by Bennetts and Flynn (2002). The effects of classroom acoustics and fluctuant conductive hearing loss for children with Downs Syndrome were stated as primary concerns for undertaking this study with four children. The researchers conducted speech-perception testing in the unamplified and amplified condition and found significant improvement in all listening situations where the sound field system was in use.

As mentioned earlier in this chapter, Updike and Conner (2003) found that students diagnosed with hearing loss, speech-language disorder, attention deficit disorder, and learning disability showed significant improvement when completing word-recognition tasks in quiet and noise under amplified and unamplified conditions.

Speech-Recognition Studies with Young Adults

Improvement in fine auditory discriminations by students in a college-level phonetics course was attributed to sound enhancement provided by an FM sound field system. In this study by Smaldino, Green, and Nelson (1997), thirty-one college students were given transcription tests both with and without the benefit of the All-Hear FM sound field system. The system was calibrated to amplify the female instructor's voice +10 dBA above the unamplified room noise level. Results showed a significant difference in the number of phonetic transcription errors made in the amplified condition compared to the unamplified listening condition. Since fewer transcription errors were made in the amplified condition, the investigators concluded that enhancing the listening environment by the use of FM sound field amplification allowed these college-age students to make maximum use of the subtle acoustic cues necessary to make fine auditory discriminations during a phonetic transcription exercise.

Speech-recognition ability of twenty young adults was assessed using the Hearing in Noise Test (HINT) presented against speech-spectrum noise under three listening conditions: (1) unaided, (2) portable FM sound field system, and (3) body-worn FM with attenuating walkman-style headphones. Crandell, Charlton, Kinder, and Kreisman (2001) designed this study to examine the perceptual benefits of the two types of FM technologies (i.e., Phonic Ear Toteable and Phonic Ear Easy Listener body-worn personal FM). The investigators used an adaptive procedure in the administration of the HINT that produced a Reception Threshold for Sentences (RTS) of 50% correct performance level. Results identified the following trends: (1) each of the FM fitting configurations produced better speech recognition than the unaided condition; (2) the body-worn FM system yielded better speech-recognition scores than the portable FM system. Use of the FM systems produced an S/N enhancement of 5.04 dB for the portable FM system and 7.91 dB for the body-worn FM system over the unaided condition. Although improvement was noted with both FM systems, the researchers suggest that for those children with greater perceptual difficulties, such as hearing loss or auditory processing disorder, a body-worn or ear-level FM system should be considered initially as the accommodation strategy due to their S/N enhancement capabilities.

Speech Recognition with Additional Sound Field Technologies

An ambitious field validation study by Lederman, Johnson, Crandell, and Smaldino (2000) showed positive effects of the SmartSpeaker "Intelligence," an adaptive signal-processing sound field system, on the speech-perception abilities of children. The adaptive signal processing is accomplished by ambient noise compensation (ANC). This study was conducted in two phases, and results from phase II will be discussed here. Participants were eighty-three children in various high-risk groups: (1) forty third-grade students with normal hearing but labeled as an at-risk group because only 21% had average or above achievement on the Colorado Student Assessment Program (CSAP); (2) twenty-one third graders identified as English Language Learners (ELL); (3) fourteen third graders receiving special education services (i.e., speech-language or learning disability); (4) nine third through fifth graders identified as hard of hearing. All testing was accomplished in the same classroom and under three S/N ratios (+6 dB, 0 dB, –6 dB). Each participant completed two listening tasks in the amplified setting under both quiet and competing noise conditions. Stimuli for the first listening task included the Word Identification Picture Intelligibility (WIPI) test (Ross & Lerman, 1979) with fifteen items at each S/N ratio. The second task was a fifty-four-item consonant-vowel (*ba, da, ga*) discrimination task, where the child was to indicate if the two syllables were the same or different. One-third of the items were administered under each of the three S/N conditions. Participants also completed a magnitude of estimation of quality (MEQ) to judge sound quality during the listening tasks. Finally, classroom teachers completed the SIFTER (Anderson, 1989). This study revealed a number of significant findings: (1) significant increase in scores occurred in five of eight conditions (WIPI at 0 and –6 S/N, same/different at –6 S/N, MEQ for both listening tasks); (2) significantly better performance by ELL students on the WIPI at all S/Ns and on both MEQs; (3) improvement on five of eight tasks by at-risk regular education students (WIPI at all S/Ns, same/different at –6 dB S/N, MEQ for word task); (4) improvement by students with hearing loss on the same/different task at –6 dB S/N; (5) SIFTER revealed problem areas for the ELL and special education groups as academics and communication and, additionally, attention for the special education group. In summary, performance was significantly improved in sixteen of forty conditions in this study using an advanced sound field technology. Use of the ANC technology produced better performance across test conditions due to its capability to sense changes in background noise levels and adjust the signal level accordingly to maintain a consistent S/N ratio.

Prendergast (2001) compared the traditional FM sound field speaker with the bending wave speaker and was able to demonstrate significantly better speech discrimination performance when using the bending wave speaker. Half-list presentations of the California Consonant Test were administered to thirty-one third-grade students and thirty-three fourth-grade students with normal hearing. The students were assessed using both the traditional and the bending wave speakers with the output set at +10 dB S/N. Results for the two listening conditions were statistically significant, with a mean score of 58.06% for the traditional speaker presentation and 65.68% for the bending wave speaker.

ATTENDING SKILLS STUDIES

Although most of the sound field FM amplification studies have been with elementary school children, Berg, Bateman, and Viehweg (1989) conducted a study in junior high school students. The effects of sound field FM amplification on attention, understanding, ease of listening, ease of teaching, and preference for the amplified listening condition were rated by students and teachers. Results showed that both groups preferred the amplified setting and that the FM equipment improved student attention and understanding as well as ease of listening and teaching. The OMNI 2001 and Realistic sound field FM amplification systems were used in this project. Interestingly, student and teacher ratings were not significantly influenced by either system.

Gilman and Danzer (1989) conducted a comprehensive math, reading, and language pre- and postassessment of second- and fourth-grade students in nine amplified and nine unamplified classrooms. The OMNI 2001 system was used in this project. Findings showed that sound field FM amplification reduced teacher voice fatigue, increased student attentiveness to verbal instruction and activities, and increased student ability to hear classroom instruction.

The effects of sound field FM amplification on a group of randomly selected, normal-hearing first- and second-grade students' on-task behavior were studied by Allen and Patton (1990). Using a systematic observation protocol, they found that under the amplified condition, students were more attentive and less distractible, and they required fewer repetitions by the teacher. In the amplified condition, a significant increase of 17% was documented for students' overall on-task behavior.

By 1990, sound field FM amplification studies of special populations other than students with known hearing loss began to emerge in the literature. The effects of amplification on attending behaviors of four- and five-year-old speech and language-delayed preschoolers were reported by Benafield (1990). The Phonic Ear Easy Listener Free Field system was installed in a language enrichment preschool classroom. Although there was no significant effect on subjects' verbalizations when using the system, there was a trend toward greater appropriate subject comments during amplified instruction. In addition, preschoolers showed an increase in several physical attending behaviors during times when sound field FM amplification was in use.

The benefit of sound field amplification on the attending skills of two groups of second-grade students was examined by Bitner, Prelock, Ellis, and Tzanis (1996). The students attended general education classes, and the groups were distinguished by their average (control group) or below-average (experimental group) performance on a selective attention task. Attention was measured using four attending behaviors (Blake, Field, Foster, Platt, & Wertz, 1991): (1) eyes turned toward the speaker, (2) body turned toward the speaker, (3) absence of extraneous body movement, and (4) absence of extraneous vocal or verbal output. The presence or absence of the four behaviors was coded in an ABAB design over four three-week periods. Use of the sound field system produced positive effects on the attending behaviors of all students. Students in the control group showed slight improvement. However, a significant increase in attending behaviors was characteristic of the experimental group, and not only did their attending skills improve, but the students were able to demonstrate the same ability to attend as the control group.

A personal desktop FM system (Audio Enhancement) was used to increase signal redundancy and auditory focus during a series of ten therapeutic sessions with five adult clients who had a variety of neurogenic disorders, including cerebral vascular accident (CVA) and traumatic brain injury (TBI). Effectiveness outcomes in this study reported by Harris and Flexer (2003) revealed improved client behaviors during both assessment and therapy sessions. Data indicated that use of the personal sound field system improved on-task attention as evidenced by a reduction in the number of redirects and by demonstration of larger gains among clients in achieving therapy outcomes.

Other studies discussed in this chapter have examined on-task behavior as part of the research design. The unanimous findings of these research efforts have been an increase in on-task behaviors when students have the benefit of sound field classroom amplification (Allcock, 1999; Allen & Patton, 1990; Benafield, 1990; Bitner, Prelock, Ellis, & Tzanis, 1996; Palmer, 1998; Rosenberg et al., 1999; Eriks-Brophy & Ayikawa, 2000; Loven, Fisk, & Johnson, 2003; Mendel, Roberts, & Walton, 2003). Refer to Table 5-4 for a summary of studies on attending, listening, and learning behaviors.

LEARNING BEHAVIOR STUDIES

Young children with early and continuing histories of hearing problems are potentially at-risk for learning. Flexer, Richards, and Buie (1993) examined teacher-perceived performance of two groups of first-grade children (N = 283) under amplified and unamplified listening conditions. Teachers were asked to note differences between the group of at-risk children (early and continuing histories of hearing problems) from a no-risk group (without known histories of hearing problems). The Screening Instrument for Targeting Educational Risk (SIFTER) (Anderson, 1989) was completed by teachers at four intervals during the school year. The SIFTER includes fifteen student-behavior statements in the areas of academics, attention, communication, class participation, and school behavior. SIFTER data showed better overall ratings for both the at-risk and no-risk groups in classrooms with sound field FM amplification. Students receiving the lowest teacher appraisal were those identified as at-risk in unamplified classrooms.

Teacher-observation rating scales have shown that the use of sound field amplification improved listening and understanding in the classroom. Baldwin and Dougherty (1997) reported that 84% of teachers (N = 19) agreed that

TABLE 5-4   Summary of sound field efficacy studies demonstrating improvement in attending, listening, and learning behaviors

Investigators	Student Population	Improvement in Attending, Listening, and Learning Behaviors Obtained with Sound Field Amplification
Berg, Bateman, & Viehweg (1989)	Regular education junior high school students	Students and teachers preferred the use of sound field amplification; students showed improved listening and understanding; and teachers noted ease of listening and teaching.
Gilman & Danzer (1989)	Nine amplified and nine control classes for second- and fourth-grade regular education students	Student attentiveness to verbal instruction and activities as well as ability to hear classroom instruction improved when using FM sound field amplification.
Allen & Patton (1990)	First- and second-grade students with normal hearing	Student distractibility and request for repetitions decreased, and on-task behavior increased significantly (17%) with sound field.
Benafield (1990)	Four- and five-year-old preschoolers with speech-language delay	Preschoolers with severe language impairment in an amplified classroom showed increased attending behaviors and improvement in the use of appropriate comments.
Flexer, Richards, & Buie (1993)	First-grade students (N = 283) with and without known history of hearing problems	Higher SIFTER scores computed for at-risk and no-risk students in amplified classes, and lowest scores were reported for at-risk students in unamplified classes.
Bitner, Prelock, Ellis, & Tzanis (1996)	Two groups of regular education second graders (attentive group and inattentive group)	Sound field amplification produced significant increase in selective attending behaviors for students with difficulty listening to instruction, particularly in the presence of noise, over four three-week periods.
Palmer (1998)	Eight kindergarten through second-grade students; single subject design	A significant decrease in inappropriate behaviors and a significant increase in appropriate behaviors were identified immediately following sound field treatment.

(continued)

TABLE 5-4 *(continued)*

Investigators	Student Population	Improvement in Attending, Listening, and Learning Behaviors Obtained with Sound Field Amplification
Allcock (1999)	Three amplified and two unamplified classrooms in New Zealand	An eight-week observation with sound field amplification (alternating two weeks on and two weeks off) found that with the amplification on, on-task behavior ranged from being 14% less on task to 50% more on task, with a mean of 18% more on-task time than when the system was off. Findings were similar for children with normal hearing and those with hearing loss.
Rosenberg et al. (1999)	ICA project (2,054 kindergarten through second-grade students in ninety-four regular education classes)	Significantly higher scores were obtained by students in amplified classes for listening, academic/ preacademic behaviors, and academic/preacademic skills, with the greatest gains for amplified kindergartners.
Eriks-Brophy & Ayukawa (2000)	Ten second- through third-grade students with hearing loss and ten age-matched peers	Significant improvements were noted in speech intelligibility scores for students with hearing loss and students with normal hearing with sound field amplification. On-task behavior improvement was noted for six of seven students when using sound field technology.
Harris & Flexer (2003)	Five adults with various neurogenic disorders (e.g., CVA, TBI)	During ten therapy sessions, attention to task improved and clients demonstrated greater gains in achieving therapy outcomes.
Loven, Fisk, & Johnson (2003)	Forty-eight students in two regular education second-grade classes	Two-way ANOVA results showed a significant interaction between room treatment and time variables, indicating increased attention for students in the amplified classroom.

sound field amplification helped their students to listen and understand better in the classroom and that their students were more attentive; 68% agreed that there was a decreased need for clarification and reinstruction following an assignment. Rosenberg et al. (1999) collected survey data from fifty-five kindergarten through second-grade general education teachers during two phases of the three-year ICA project and found high levels of agreement from teachers that (1) the need to repeat directions and information decreased (96–100%), (2) students seemed to listen and understand better (92–93%), (3) students were more attentive (93–100%), and (4) sound field amplification helped with classroom control and behavior management (80–86%).

Palmer (1998) reported on the ecobehavioral impact of sound field amplification through a systematic investigation of the impact of initiation and removal of the sound reinforcement technology on observable classroom behaviors. This single-subject design involved observations of eight children in four classrooms (one kindergarten, two first grades, and one second grade). This ambitious study was conducted over a two-year period, with data collection occurring for kindergarten students in the first year and for the first and second graders in the following year. Amplification was provided using the Omni 2000 and the Phonic Ear sound field systems with a three-speaker arrangement; a +6 to +10 dB S/N was achieved. This investigator used the Code for Instructional Structure and Student Achievement Response (CISSAR) (Greenwood, Schulte, Kohler, Dinwiddie, & Carta, 1986) for data collection, as it allows for an observer to record ecobehavioral interaction data observed in the classroom. Task management and competing or inappropriate responses by students, as well as teacher position and behavior, were observed. Findings of this study showed that the introduction of sound field amplification reduced competing and inappropriate behaviors and increased the occurrence of task management for each of the students. Sound field amplification did not affect teacher behavior or position, and as such, Palmer concluded that changes in student behavior were related to the amplified listening condition. These findings corroborate the results obtained by Flexer et al. (1994) in support of a decrease in competing or inappropriate behaviors during the use of sound field amplification. In addition, teachers wished to continue using the sound field technology due to its benefits related to either task management or competing or inappropriate behaviors (i.e., reduced vocal fatigue, reduced need for repetitions, decreased transition time, increased student attention, increased control of the class.)

The Improving Classroom Acoustics (ICA) three-year project was designed to examine improvement in listening behaviors, academic/preacademic behaviors, and academic/preacademic skills for early-grade students (kindergarten through second grade) when using sound field amplification (Rosenberg et al., 1999). This special project, funded by the Florida Department of Education, Division of Public Schools, and the Bureau of Education for Exceptional Students through federal assistance under the Individuals with Disabilities Education Act (IDEA), Part B, involved 2,054 students in ninety-four general education classrooms in thirty-three elementary schools in Florida. For this two-phase study, the four-speaker Phonic Ear Easy Listener Free Field system was installed in sixty-four experimental (amplified) classrooms and thirty control (unamplified) classrooms. The study also included unoccupied and occupied classroom noise measurements, which were not different than previously reported studies (Crandell, 1991; Finitzo-Heiber & Tillman, 1978). Teachers in experimental classrooms showed an average gain in vocal intensity of +6.94 dB(A).

In Phase I of the ICA project, 855 students in sixty classrooms were observed prior to use of sound field amplification and at six- and twelve-week intervals during use, and 804 students were also observed at twenty-one and thirty weeks during use. In Phase II, 735 students in thirty-four classrooms were observed prior to use of sound field amplification and four weeks following its removal. Teachers completed the Listening and Learning Observation (LLO) form devised for this project. Ten randomly selected students in each class were also observed using an adaptation of the Evaluation of Classroom Listening Behaviors (ECLB) (VanDyke, 1985). Results showed that students in amplified classrooms demonstrated a significantly greater change in listening behaviors, academic/preacademic behaviors, and academic/pre-academic skills, and at a faster rate than their peers in unamplified classrooms. In addition, the greatest gains were made by younger students in amplified classrooms. Results from the LLO and the ECLB showed the same trend.

ICA project evaluation showed overwhelming support from students, teachers, parents, and administrators toward use of sound field FM amplification. When asked if they wanted to use the listening equipment again next year, 94% of the students responded affirmatively. Teachers used the systems an average of 3.88 to 4.38 hours per day, and all of the teachers agreed that decreased vocal strain was their primary benefit from using the sound field FM amplification system. Between 24.5% and 38% of the parents who completed the evaluation form observed the FM system in operation. Parents gave their highest rating to the item requesting that their child be able to use the sound field FM amplification system again next year. Administrators acknowledged that class instruction and management appeared to be enhanced when teachers used classroom amplification and also commented that it helped to "save the teacher's voices."

DiSarno, Schowalter, and Grassa (2002) conducted a study with high school students to determine the effect of teacher bias on the results of classroom amplification use. The study involved a two-member team teaching arrangement in a multiage classroom (ninth through twelfth grades) for nine students with learning disabilities. A Phonic Ear wireless four-speaker FM sound field system was installed for the three-month study. The Listening and

Learning Observation (LLO) and an adaptation of the Evaluation of Classroom Listening Behaviors (ECLB) were completed independently by both teachers prior to using the sound field system and again following six and twelve weeks of use. Findings indicated a significant improvement in the listening and academic behaviors of these students with learning disabilities after using the classroom amplification for twelve weeks. The teachers also indicated that the primary benefits they noted from using the sound field amplification were (1) an increase in the teacher's ability to gain and maintain students' attention, and (2) a decrease in teacher vocal strain and fatigue.

When the Audio Enhancement infrared sound field systems were installed in all of Florida's Ocoee Middle School classrooms as part of the SMART (Soundly Made, Accountable, Reasonable and Thrifty) school of the future project, the principal noted a 40% decline in discipline incidents over a one-year period. Sound field amplification, at least in part, contributed to the students' increased opportunities to focus and remain on task (Rittner-Heir, 2001). Anecdotal comments from students, teachers, parents, and administrators also support the benefits of this listening enhancement technology.

TEACHER RESPONSE TO SOUND FIELD FM AMPLIFICATION

This section will examine various teacher responses to, and benefits derived from, sound field amplification.

Teacher Preference for Sound Field Technology

Teacher response to sound field FM amplification in the classroom has been overwhelming once they have had the opportunity to use this equipment, even on a limited basis. A teacher survey conducted by Allen (1993) showed that teachers who have experience using sound field FM systems in their classrooms value it over eight other types of instructional delivery equipment such as overhead projectors, televisions, computers, VCRs, CD-ROMs, and filmstrip projectors. When a group of thirty teachers with at least three days of experience using sound field FM amplification systems rated their first choice of instructional delivery equipment, sound field FM amplification systems received 34% of the top choices, followed by overhead projectors (18%) and computers (16%). Interestingly, two additional groups of teachers, one with indirect exposure to sound field amplification and the other with no exposure to this equipment, rated the overhead projector as their top choice.

Vocal Health Benefits

After several weeks' experience, sound field amplification was evaluated by twenty early-grade teachers (kindergarten through third grade) in traditional and open pod classrooms in Rochester, Minnesota. The Phonic Ear Easy Listener Free Field system was used for this study by Nelson and Schmidt (1993). They obtained feedback using a devised teacher questionnaire and found that teachers in the open classroom environments realized greater success in using the sound field technology than did those teachers in traditional classrooms. Teachers also identified improvement in ease of classroom control, student attentiveness (and subsequent decrease in the need for repetitions), as well as decreased vocal strain and fatigue.

Vocal health is a common concern among classroom teachers and school administrators. Allen (1995) reported that approximately 56% of 141 elementary teachers in Dubuque, Iowa, indicated at least one episode of vocal abuse or fatigue during the school year. The 60% of the teachers who had never had the benefit of using sound field amplification estimated that they took an estimated 9.7 sick days per year due to vocal maladies. On the other hand, 40% of the teachers with experience using sound field amplification estimated that when they were without this technology, they averaged .93 sick days per year due to vocal health issues, but when whey were using the systems their use of sick days for vocal-related problems was reduced to an average .34 days per teacher. While this data supports the use of sound field amplification as a means to preserve teachers' vocal health, it also suggests that the use of sound field amplification could produce a substantial cost-saving benefit for the school district.

Sapienza, Crandell, and Curtis (1999) studied the effects of sound field amplification on a group of ten classroom teachers. They examined the effectiveness of sound field amplification as a strategy to reduce the sound pressure level (SLP) of the teachers' voices during classroom instruction. The study was conducted during classroom lectures both with and without the benefit of sound field amplification. Findings showed that this technology can reduce the teacher's overall speech volume, which in turn can limit the potential for vocal health problems such as vocal fatigue and hoarseness. The results indicated that when using the sound field amplification, teachers demonstrated a significant 2.42 dB decrease in SPL.

In a single-subject design experiment, English, Kasper, and Grunberg (2003) assessed vocal characteristic information from a female college professor when she was lecturing both with and without sound field amplification. A Phonic Ear Easy Listener four-speaker sound field system was used in this study, which was designed to establish a relationship between teaching in acoustically poor conditions and vocal parameters correlating to vocal disturbance. Before and after class, the instructor provided a voice sample for purposes of evaluating frequency, harmonic-to-noise (H/N) ratio, jitter percent, and shimmer (dB). Results showed a significant increase in jitter (i.e., cycle-to-cycle changes in frequency) when teaching without the benefit of sound field amplification, but jitter did not increase significantly when using the technology.

Table 5-5 provides a summary of teacher-related benefits from using sound field amplification. Several studies have revealed, primarily through teacher survey or informal data gathering, that teachers find sound field amplification to reduce vocal strain and fatigue (Osborn, VonderEmbse, & Graves, 1989; Nelson & Schmidt, 1993; Baldwin & Dougherty, 1997; Palmer, 1998; Valente, 1998; Rosenberg et al., 1999; Dairi, 2000; Eriks-Brophy & Ayukawa, 2000; Long & Flexer, 2001; DiSarno, Schowalter, & Grassa, 2002; Mendel, Roberts, & Walton, 2003).

Cost-Effectiveness

Three studies have reported on the cost-effectiveness benefit of sound field amplification, while others have speculated on the benefits of the long-term effects of the investment in this classroom sound enhancement technology. Osborn, VonderEmsbe, and Graves (1989) stated that the initial implementation costs at that time, approximately $1,700 per classroom, was easily supported as being far more cost-effective than the annual cost of $2,600 to educate a child in a special education classroom. The MARRS study noted that students in amplified classrooms show significant academic gain at a faster rate, to a higher level, and at one-tenth the cost of students in a resource-room setting (Ray, 1987). Rosenberg (1998) compared two newly constructed portable classrooms; one was acoustically modified for students with hearing loss, and the other received sound field amplification as an accommodation. The sound field system was provided as an alternative accommodation at less than one-fourth the cost of the construction modifications in the specially modified portable classroom. The Improving Classroom Acoustics Project also studied the cost-effectiveness of sound field amplification when compared to other frequently used types of instructional delivery equipment. The per-person daily cost for a typical class (i.e., twenty-five students, one teacher) was estimated at $.14 to $.16. When a five-year longevity factor was added, the daily cost decreased to $.03 per person. Refer to Table 5-6 for a summary of these studies.

SUMMARY

Many of these studies found that younger children tended to exhibit greater behavior changes and academic growth than did older children. This may be attributable in part to the fact that younger children are often plagued by such problems as otitis media and require speech to be louder in order to hear clearly (Crandell & Smaldino, 1992; Flexer, 1992). Collectively, results of sound field amplification research suggest significant benefits for students in the areas of literacy and academic achievement, speech-recognition enhancement in quiet and noise, and on-task behavior related to attentional

TABLE 5-5   Summary of sound field efficacy studies demonstrating teacher preferences and benefits from the use of sound field amplification

Investigators	Population	Results Obtained with Sound Field Amplification	Preferences and Benefits
Allen (1993)	Ninety general education elementary teachers	Once familiar with the system, teachers ranked sound field's usefulness above other instructional delivery equipment.	Preference
Nelson & Schmidt (1993)	Twenty general education-K–3 teachers	Teachers in open classrooms reported greater success than those in traditional classrooms, although all teachers identified benefits.	Open classroom
Osborn, Vonder Embse, & Graves (1989)	Forty-seven amplified K–3 regular education classrooms	Fewer teacher absences due to fatigue and laryngitis when using sound field amplification	Teacher's voice
Baldwin & Dougherty (1997)	Nineteen general education elementary classroom teachers	Sound field helped to reduce emotional strain and vocal fatigue (79%)	Teacher's voice
Rosenberg et al. (1999)	Fifty-five general education K–2 teachers	Teachers agreed 100% that reduced vocal strain was the greatest benefit from sound field amplification.	Teacher's voice
Sapienza, Crandell, & Curtis (1999)	Ten classroom teachers	Using sound field amplification, teachers showed a significant 2.42 dB decrease in SPL during classroom instruction.	Vocal hygiene
English, Kasper, & Grunberg (2003)	Single-subject design (female college instructor)	Results showed a significant increase in jitter (i.e., cycle-to-cycle changes in frequency) when teaching without the benefit of sound field amplification but no significant increase in jitter when using the technology.	Vocal health
Mendel, Roberts, & Walton (2003)	Seven kindergarten and first-grade teachers; two-year longitudinal study	Survey indicated 95% positive response, indicating universal support for use of sound field amplification in kindergarten and first-grade classrooms.	Teacher evaluation

TABLE 5-6   Summary of sound field efficacy studies demonstrating cost-effectiveness of sound field amplification

Investigators	Population	Cost-Effectiveness of Sound Field Amplification
Sarff (1981); Ray, Sarff, and Glassford (1984)	MARRS project (fourth-through sixth-grade students with minimal hearing loss, academic deficit, and normal learning potential)	The MARRS project demonstrated that students with minimal hearing loss and learning disabilities in amplified classrooms made significant academic gains at a faster rate, to a higher level, and at one-tenth the cost of students in unamplified resource-room settings.
Rosenberg (1998)	One acoustically modified and one amplified relocatable classroom	Sound field amplification was provided at one-fourth the cost of acoustical modifications in newly constructed relocatable classrooms.
Rosenberg et al. (1999)	Fifty-four general education K–2 amplified classrooms	Typical classroom (twenty-five students, one teacher) daily cost per person was $.14 or $.03 per day over five years.

skills and learning behaviors. Students, teachers, parents, and school administrators have indicated positive approval for the use of sound field technology in classrooms.

Additional research on the efficacy of sound field amplification is needed in the following areas in order to continue to promote the value of this technology: longitudinal literacy-based studies; special populations (e.g., auditory processing disorder, learning disability, language-impairment, attention deficit disorder); general population from preschool through geriatric ages (e.g., common use areas in assisted living facilities); microphone and speaker technologies; and other innovative sound field technology options.

As the potential market for sound field amplification continues to grow, the need for ongoing research is evident. Audiologists can enhance the credibility of the benefits of sound field amplification by applying the principles of evidence-based practice (EBP) when designing, conducting, and analyzing data from research studies designed to evaluate the effectiveness of this technology. Further, using EPB principles to design sound field amplification research studies is a proactive means to support inclusion of this technology as a necessary component of universal classroom design. Audiologists must maintain their leadership role in promoting the concept and benefits of sound field amplification not only as a means of helping students with known hearing loss but also as a prevention and intervention strategy to provide all students with enhanced access to acoustic signals in their listening and learning environments.

DISCUSSION TOPICS

1. Explain the different sound field amplification system options that have been studied.
2. Based on efficacy studies, what are the major effects of a sound field amplification system on literacy and academic achievement?
3. Briefly describe the positive effects of sound field amplification on speech-recognition performance in these categories:

   - distance from the speaker
   - general education classrooms
   - listeners with hearing loss
   - listeners with cochlear implants
   - other special needs populations
   - young adults
   - innovative sound field technologies

4. What effect does sound field amplification have on attending skills? What are the attending skills and populations that have been studied?
5. Explain the findings of studies examining the effects of sound field amplification on learning in children.
6. How have teachers responded to use of sound field amplification in the classroom? Why?
7. Explain the vocal health benefits that result from use of sound field amplification.
8. Why is the use of sound field amplification seen as cost-effective?

REFERENCES

Allcock, J. (1999). Report of FM soundfield study: Paremata School 1997. Study funded by the Oticon Foundation, available at http://www.oticon.org.nz/pdf/OTICONParamataresearchreport.pdf.

Allen, L. (1993). Promoting the usefulness of classroom amplification equipment. *Educational Audiology Monograph, 3,* 32–34.

Allen, L. (1995). The effect of sound-field amplification on teacher vocal abuse problems. Paper presented at the Educational Audiology Association Conference, Lake Lure, NC.

Allen, L., & Patton, D. (1990, November). Effects of sound field amplification on students' on-task behavior. Paper presented at the American Speech-Language-Hearing convention, Seattle, WA.

Anderson, K. (1989). *Screening instrument for targeting educational risk (SIFTER)*. Tampa, FL: Educational Audiology Association.

Anderson, K. (1999). Sound field FM use by children with severe hearing loss: Two case studies. *Journal of Educational Audiology, 7*, 54–57.

Anderson, K., & Smaldino, J. (1998). *The listening inventories for education (LIFE)*. Tampa, FL: Educational Audiology Association.

Baldwin, D., & Dougherty, C. (1997). A Montana experience with classroom amplification. *Journal of Educational Audiology, 5*, 44–46.

Benafield, N. (1990). The effects of sound field amplification on the attending behaviors of speech and language-delayed preschool children. Unpublished master's thesis, University of Arkansas at Little Rock.

Bennetts, L., & Flynn, M. (2002). Improving the classroom listening skills of children with Down syndrome by using sound-field amplification. *Down Syndrome Research and Practice, 8*(1), 19–24.

Berg, F., Bateman, R., & Viehweg, S. (1989, November). Sound field FM amplification in junior high school classrooms. Paper presented at the American Speech-Language-Hearing Association convention, St. Louis, MO.

Bitner, B., Prelock, P., Ellis, C., & Tzanis, E. (1996, November). Group sound field amplification and attending behaviors in the classroom setting. Paper presented at the American Speech-Language-Hearing convention, Seattle, WA.

Blair, J., Myrup, C., & Viehweg, S. (1989). Comparison of the effectiveness of hard-of-hearing children using three types of amplification. *Educational Audiology Monograph, 1*, 48–55.

Blake, R., Field, C., Platt, F., & Wertz, P. (1991). Effect of FM auditory trainers on attending behaviors of learning disabled children. *Language, Speech, and Hearing Services in the Schools, 21*, 177–182.

Bourque, M. L., & Byrd, S. (Eds.). (2000, November). Student performance standards on the national assessment of educational progress: Affirmations and improvements. Washington, DC: National Assessment Governing Board. Available at http://www.nagb.org/pubs/studentperfstandard.pdf.

Crandell, C. (1991). The effects of classroom amplification on children with normal hearing: Implications for intervention strategies. *Educational Audiology Monograph, 2*, 18–38.

Crandell, C. (1993). A comparison of commercially-available frequency modulation sound field amplification systems. *Educational Audiology Monograph, 3*, 15–20.

Crandell, C. (1996). Effects of sound-field FM amplification on the speech perception of ESL children. *Educational Audiology Monograph, 4*, 1–5.

Crandell, C., & Bess, F. (1986, November). Sound-field amplification in the classroom setting. Paper presented at the American Speech-Language-Hearing Association convention, New Orleans, LA.

Crandell, C., Charlton, M., Kinder, M., & Kreisman, B. (2001). Effects of portable sound field FM systems on speech perception in noise. *Journal of Educational Audiology, 9*, 8–12.

Crandell, C., Holmes, A., Flexer, C., & Payne, M. (1998). Effects of sound field FM amplification on the speech recognition of listeners with cochlear implants. *Journal of Educational Audiology, 6*, 21–27.

Crandell, C., & Smaldino, J. (1992). Sound-field amplification in the classroom. *American Journal of Audiology, 1*(4), 16–18.

Crandell, C., & Smaldino, J. (1996). Speech perception in noise by children for whom English is a second language. *American Journal of Audiology, 5*, 47–51.

Crandell, C., & Smaldino, J. (2000). Current practices in classroom sound field FM amplification. *Journal of Educational Audiology, 8,* 9–17.

Crandell, C., Smaldino, J., & Flexer, C. (1995). *Sound-field FM amplification: Theory and practical applications.* Clifton Park, NY: Thomson Delmar Learning.

Dairi, B. (2000). Using sound field FM systems to improve literacy scores. *Advance for Speech-Language Pathologists and Audiologists, 10*(27), 5, 13.

DiSarno, N., Schowalter, M., & Grassa, P. (2002). Classroom amplification to enhance student performance. *Teaching Exceptional Children, 34*(6), 20–25.

English, K., Kasper, S., & Grunberg, Z. (2003). Sound field amplification and the teaching voice. Available at http://www.speechpathology.com/articles/arc_disp.asp?id=1.

Eriks-Brophy, A., & Ayukawa, H. (2000). The benefits of sound field amplification in classrooms of Inuit students of Nunavik: A pilot project. *Language, Speech, and Hearing Services in Schools, 31,* 324–335.

Finitzo-Heiber, T., & Tillman, T. (1978). Room acoustic effects on monosyllabic word discrimination ability for normal and hearing impaired children. *Journal of Speech and Hearing Research, 21,* 440–448.

Flexer, C. (1989). Turn on sound: An odyssey of sound field amplification. *Educational Audiology Association Newsletter, 5*(5), 6–7.

Flexer C. (1992). Classroom public address systems. In M. Ross, (Ed.), *FM auditory training systems: Characteristics, selection & use* (pp. 189–209). Timonium, MD: York Press.

Flexer, C. (2002). Rationale and use of sound field systems: An update. *The Hearing Journal, 55*(8), 10–18.

Flexer, C., Biley, K., Hinkley, A., Harkema, C., & Holcomb, J. (2002). Using sound-field systems to teach phonemic awareness to pre-schoolers. *The Hearing Journal, 55*(3), 38–44.

Flexer, C., Millin, J., & Brown, L. (1990). Children with developmental disabilities: The effect of sound field amplification on word identification. *Language, Speech and Hearing Services in Schools, 21,* 177–182.

Flexer, C., Richards, C., & Buie, C. (1993, April). Soundfield amplification for regular kindergarten and first grade classrooms: A longitudinal study of fluctuating hearing loss and pupil performance. Paper presented at the American Academy of Audiology convention, Phoenix, AZ.

Gilman, L., & Danzer, V. (1989, November). Use of FM sound field amplification in regular classrooms. Paper presented at the American Speech-Language-Hearing Association convention, St. Louis, MO.

Gordon-Langbein, A., & Metinger, M. (1999). Using audio systems in schools. *Media and Methods Magazine.*

Greenwood, C., Schulte, D., Kohler, F., Dinwiddie, G., & Carta, J. (1986). Assessment and analysis of ecobehavioral interaction in school settings. In R. J. Prinz (Ed.), *Advances in behavioral assessment of children and families* (pp. 69–98). Lincoln, NE: JAI Press.

Harris, N., & Flexer, C. (2003). Adults with neurogenic disorders: Enhancing treatment with a desktop amplifier. Poster presentation at the American Speech-Language-Hearing Association Annual Convention, Chicago, IL.

Howell, P. (1996). Effects of sound-field amplification on test scores of normally hearing children in a regular education classroom. Unpublished manuscript.

Irwin, S., Kirsch, A. J., Jenkins, L., and Kolstad, A. (1993). *Adult literacy in America: A first look at the findings of the National Adult Literacy Survey.* Washington, DC: National Center for Education Statistics.

Jones, J., Berg, F., & Viehweg, S. (1989). Listening of kindergarten students under close, distant, and sound field FM amplification conditions. *Educational Audiology Monograph, 1*, 56–65.

Kirsch, I. S., Jungeblut, A., Jenkins, L., & Kolstad, A. (1993). *Adult literacy in America: A first look at the results of the National Adult Literacy Survey* (Publication NCES 93275). Washington, DC: National Center for Education Statistics. Available at http://nces.ed.gov/pubsearch/pubsinfo.asp?pubid=93275.

Lederman, N., Johnson, C., Crandell, C., & Smaldino, J. (2000). The development and validation of an "intelligent" classroom sound field frequency modulation (FM) system. *Journal of Educational Audiology, 8*, 37–42.

Levitt, H., & Ross, M. (2002). Developments in research and technology: Hearing-assistive technologies. *Volta Voices, 9*(2), 7–8.

Long, S., & Flexer, C. (2001). Sound field amplification for all. *Advance for Speech-Language Pathologists and Audiologists, 11*(27), 10–11.

Loven, F., Fisk, K., & Johnson, S. (2003). Classroom amplification systems on early academic achievement and attention. Poster session presentation at the American Speech-Language-Hearing Association Annual Convention, Chicago, IL.

Massie, R. (2003). The impact of sound field amplification in mainstream classrooms. Paper presented at the Australia and New Zealand Conference for Educators of the Deaf, Fremantle, WA.

McCarty, P., & Gertel, S. (2003). Designing the best learning environments to maximize student performance. Presentation at the Council of Educational Facility Planners International Convention, Chicago, IL.

Mendel, L., Roberts, R., & Walton, J. (2003). Speech perception benefits from sound field FM amplification. *American Journal of Audiology, 12*, 114–124.

Moog, J., & Geers, A. (1990) Early speech perception (ESP) test for profoundly hearing-impaired children. St. Louis, MO: Central Institute for the Deaf.

Mills, M. (1991). A practical look at classroom amplification. *Educational Audiology Monograph, 2*(1), 39–42.

Nelson, D., & Schmidt, M. (1993). Take anything else, but leave my classroom FM system! *Perspectives, 12*(1), 8–11.

Neuss, D., Blair, J., & Viehweg, S. (1991). Sound field amplification: Does it improve word recognition in a background of noise for students with minimal hearing impairments? *Educational Audiology Monograph, 2*, 43–52.

Nilsson, M., Soli, S. D., & Sullivan, J. (1994). Development of the Hearing in Noise Test for the measurement of speech reception thresholds in quiet and in noise. *Journal of the Acoustical Society of America, 95*, 1085–1099.

Osborn, J., VonderEmbse, D., & Graves, L. (1989). Development of a model program using sound field amplification for prevention of auditory-based learning disabilities. Unpublished study, Putnam County Office of Education, Ottawa, OH.

Palmer, C. (1998). Quantification of the ecobehavioral impact of a soundfield system. *Journal of Speech, Language, and Hearing Research, 41*(4), 819–833.

Poissant, S., Brackett, D., & Maxon, A. (1998). Cochlear implant users listening in noise: Benefits of sound field amplification. *Educational Audiology Review, 15*(1), 3.

Prendergast, S. (2001). A comparison of the performance of classroom amplification with traditional and bending wave speakers. *Journal of Educational Audiology, 9*, 1–6.

Ray, H. (1987, Spring). Put a microphone on the teacher: A simple solution for the difficult problems of mild hearing loss. *The Clinical Connection,* 14–15.

Ray, H. (1992). *Summary of MARRS adoption data validated in 1992.* Norris City, IL: Wabash and Ohio Special Education District.

Ray, H., Sarff, L. S., & Glassford, J. E. (1984, Summer/Fall). Sound field amplification: An innovative educational intervention for mainstreamed learning disabled students. *The Directive Teacher,* 18–20.

Rittner-Heir, R. (2001). Sounds like a winner. *School Planning & Management, 40*(1), 92–94.

Rosenberg, G. (1998). Relocatable classrooms: Acoustical modifications or FM sound field classroom amplification? *Journal of Educational Audiology, 6,* 9–13.

Rosenberg, G., Blake-Rahter, P., Heavner, J., Allen, L., Redmond, B., Phillips, J., & Stigers, K. (1999). Improving classroom acoustics (ICA): A three-year FM sound field classroom amplification study. *Journal of Educational Audiology, 7,* 8–28.

Ross, M., & Lerman, J. (1979). A picture identification test for hearing-impaired children. *Journal of Speech and Hearing Research, 13,* 44–53.

Sapienza, C., Crandell, C., & Curtis, B. (1999). Effects of sound-field frequency modulation amplification on reducing teachers' sound pressure level in the classroom. *Journal of Voice, 13,* 375–381.

Sarff, L. (1981). An innovative use of free-field amplification in classrooms. In R. Roeser & M. Downs (Eds.), *Auditory disorders in school children* (pp. 263–272). New York: Thieme-Stratton.

Sarff, L., Ray, H., & Bagwell, C., (1981). Why not amplification in every classroom? *Hearing Aid Journal, 34*(10), 11, 47–52.

Schermer, D. (1991). Briggs sound amplified classroom study. Unpublished study, Briggs Elementary School, Maquoketa, IA.

Smaldino, J., Green, D., & Nelson, G. (1997). The effects of sound-field amplification on fine auditory discrimination. *Educational Audiology Monograph, 5,* 29–31.

Torgesen, J., & Bryant, B. (1994). *Test of phonological awareness.* Austin, TX: Pro-Ed.

Updike, C., & Conner, K. (2003, November). Classroom amplification and its impact on auditory discrimination. Poster session presentation at the American Speech-Language-Hearing Association Annual Convention, Chicago, IL.

U.S. Department of Education (2001). National Center for Education Statistics: National Assessment of Educational Progress (NAEP), 1992–2000 Reading Assessments, Washington, DC.

Valente, M. (1998). Effects of sound field amplification upon academic performance in college students. *Journal of Educational Audiology, 6,* 14–20.

VanDyke, J. (1985). Evaluating amplification in the classroom. *Rocky Mountain Journal of Communication Disorders, 1,* 7–9.

Yopp, H. (1995). A test for assessing phonemic awareness in young children. *Reading Teacher, 49*(1), 20–29.

Zabel, H., & Tabor, M. (1993). Effects of classroom amplification on spelling performance of elementary school children. *Educational Audiology Monograph, 3,* 5–9.

PRACTICAL APPLICATIONS OF SOUND FIELD AMPLIFICATION

CHAPTER 6

Classroom Acoustic Measurements

Joseph J. Smaldino, PhD
Carl C. Crandell, PhD
Brian M. Kreisman, PhD

KEY POINTS

- Observation of the classroom should occur prior to acoustic modifications.
- Reverberation time and noise are important determinants for speech perception.
- Reverberation time can be measured via various hardware and software devices or estimated with different formulae.
- Noise can be measured via a sound-level meter.
- Noise criteria and room criteria curves can be established to determine the effects of noise on speech perception in the classroom.
- Steps for preparation of acoustical recommendations for a classroom are provided.

A typical classroom is an active environment that continually changes from one learning activity to another. For this reason, acoustical environments of classrooms are often difficult to measure because acoustical parameters change as a function of time. For example, intensity variations in the teacher's voice and the ambient noise levels in the classroom continually alter the signal-to-noise (S/N) ratio. Likewise, speaker-to-listener distances vary as the teacher (and students) move around the classroom. Therefore, an understanding of the status and dynamics of a particular classroom must be understood before measurements, and subsequent changes, in the acoustical environment can be considered. This chapter will discuss methods of measuring the classroom acoustical environment. Specifically, methods of measuring and estimating reverberation time and noise in a classroom will be addressed, along with steps for developing recommendations for a classroom.

CLASSROOM OBSERVATION

The most direct manner by which to gain an understanding of the dynamics is to observe the room during a part of the school day with the teacher and students in the room. It is likely that many classroom configurations are used throughout the school day. Hence, each teaching configuration must be considered separately when determining the acoustics of the classroom. Otherwise, measurements obtained for one condition (i.e., the teacher speaking from the front of the room) may not accurately reflect other conditions, such as small student groups with the teacher walking around the classroom. The first step in obtaining acoustic measurements for a classroom is to determine the location of the teacher and students when the majority of instruction takes place. This step includes documenting the distances between the teacher and students as well as the distances between individual students. In addition, the audiologist should be aware of obvious sources of background noise, any disabilities (such as hearing loss or auditory processing disorders) that the children may have, teaching style, and additional types of technology in the room. Recording observations and measurements for each classroom is helpful.

REVERBERATION MEASUREMENTS IN THE CLASSROOM

Recall from earlier chapters that the sound of a teacher's voice traveling to a student's ears has three distinct components. Those components are direct sound, early reflections, and reverberation. The direct sound travels from the teacher to the student without reflecting off any surfaces within the room. Because the direct sound goes directly to the listener, it is the first sound to reach the student's ears. Reflected sounds are those sounds that bounce off one or more room surfaces on their way to the listener. Reflected sounds that arrive at the listener's ear within fifty milliseconds are usually considered to be early, or first-order, reflections. Reflected sounds are measured via a spectrum analyzer. A spectrum analyzer displays the intensity spectrum level (ISL). The ISL is the spectral frequency density expressed in decibels and can be described by the following equation:

$$\text{ISL}(f) = [I_f(f) \times 1\text{Hz}]/I_{ref} \tag{6.1}$$

where I_{ref} is the reference intensity of ten to twelve Pascals. Early reflections generally strike only one surface in the room before reaching the listener's ears and cannot be distinguished from direct sound. Because they cannot be distinguished from direct sound, early reflections actually combine with the direct sound to increase the perceived loudness of the signal (Bradley, 1986; Lochner & Burger, 1964). An increase in the loudness of a signal has been demonstrated to increase speech perception (Nabelek & Nabelek, 1994).

Reverberation refers to the persistence or prolongation of sound as sound waves reflect off hard surfaces (e.g., walls, ceilings, floors, desks, etc.) within an environment. Reverberation time is often measured by the time it takes for a sound, at a specific frequency, to decrease 60 dB below its initial level (or one-millionth of its original intensity) following termination of the signal (Bolt & MacDonald, 1949; Lochner & Burger, 1964; Knudsen & Harris, 1978; Kurtovic, 1975). This is referred to as RT_{60}. A number of factors affect RT. Such factors include (1) the dimensions, volume, and shape of the room; and (2) the types and surface areas of absorptive and reflective materials in the room.

Reverberation time is an important determinant for speech perception. For adults with normal hearing, speech perception is not compromised until the RT exceeds approximately 1.0 second (Crum, 1974; Gelfand & Silman, 1979; Nabelek & Pickett, 1974a, 1974b). In contrast, speech perception for listeners with SNHL is reduced when the RT exceeds approximately 0.4–0.5 seconds (Crandell, 1991a, 1991b, 1992; Crandell & Bess, 1986). For example, Finitzo-Hieber and Tillman (1978) examined the effect of room acoustics on the monosyllabic word perception of twelve children with normal hearing and twelve children with hearing impairment. Three reverberation times (0.0, 0.4, and 1.2 seconds) were studied. Data indicated that without noise competition (signal-to-noise ratio = ¥), children with normal hearing obtained speech-perception scores of 94.5%, 92.5%, and 76.5% for the 0.0-, 0.4-, and 1.2-second listening conditions, respectively. Under the same conditions, the group of children with hearing impairment obtained speech-perception scores of 87.5%, 69.0%, and 61.8%.

Unfortunately, assessing the effects of speech perception on reverberation in the clinical setting is difficult due to the expense of the test room that can be acoustically modified in order to change reverberation time and the time needed to change conditions. Of course, speech perception can be assessed in real-world environments that contain reverberation. Classroom reverberation can also be simulated via models produced using computer-aided design (CAD) or via hardware-based reverberation simulators. CAD allows the construction of a model of a three-dimensional room. The ceiling, walls, floor, and furnishings of the room are drawn to scale, and text files are created that contain absorption and diffusion coefficients for the various surfaces. The CAD model can then be imported into other computer programs, such as the Computer Aided Theater Technique (CATT) CATT-Acoustic program. Software such as CATT-Acoustic allows the creation of a virtual room in which the acoustic characteristics, including RT, can be changed. Simulated reverberation programs are commonly used for architectural design. Such programs are critical in the design stage for building or remodeling rooms because they enable the user to determine the sound quality of the room with different acoustic modifications, without physically making changes to the room. Rather, it is only necessary to change the absorption and diffusion characteristics for a particular surface to hear the effect of the change produced through the simulation program. For example, the change in speech-perception sound quality for carpeted floors, instead of tile floors, can be determined relatively quickly by substituting different absorption and diffusion characteristics. Computer programs that simulate reverberation are employed in the design of concert halls in order to determine the sound quality of music in that environment.

Reverberation also can be simulated via hardware-based reverberation simulators. One such instrument, the Lexicon MPX-550 Effects Processor, is a dual-channel processor. One channel consists of reverberation algorithms, while the other channel consists of delay algorithms. The MPX-550 has 240 preprogrammed settings with reverberation algorithms such as room, chamber, plate, gate, hall, and ambiance. User-customized programs contain up to eight adjustable parameters. Reverberation characteristics can be adjusted via delay, pitch, and modulation effects. Hardware-based reverberation simulators often are employed in recording studios and as speaker delays for amplifying large auditoriums.

To date, there remains a paucity of data demonstrating the effect of simulated reverberation on speech perception in listeners with normal hearing or hearing impairment. Thus, it is not known whether any of the simulations can approximate the speech perception attained in actual rooms. At present, only one investigation has attempted to examine the effects of simulated reverberation on speech perception (Nabelek & Robinette, 1978). This investigation used the Modified Rhyme Test (MRT) to assess speech perception in reverberation and noise. In their first experiment, subjects consisted of five adults with normal hearing and seven adults with hearing impairment. Multitalker babble served as the noise competition. Two different RTs, 0.25 to 0.50 second (measured in actual rooms), were assessed. This range of actual room RTs caused a significant deterioration in speech-perception scores in both groups. Specifically, in the binaural condition, subjects with normal hearing obtained speech-perception scores of 67.5% and 56.3% for the 0.25- and 0.50-second listening conditions, respectively. Under the same conditions, subjects with hearing impairment obtained speech-perception scores of 69.0% and 45.7%. The trend of the data indicated that as hearing loss increased, the reverberation effect decreased. Five subjects with normal hearing and five subjects with hearing impairment participated in the second experiment. In this experiment, a simulated reverberation was produced via a PDP-12 computer system. The computer was programmed to act as a multiple delay line, with the direct sound followed by five distinct reflections. Three different simulated RTs were assessed: 0.17, 0.44, and 0.61 second. Results indicated that with the computer-programmed simulated reverberation, no significant changes in speech-perception scores were noted. Neither the difference between the mean scores of the normal-hearing and hearing-impaired groups (66.5% and 63.9%, respectively) nor the differences between mean scores for the three RTs (66.0%, 63.7%, and 65.9% for 0.17, 0.44, and 0.61 second, respectively), were statistically significant. In other words, the simulated reverberation did not emulate the actual room reverberation.

We are conducting an investigation to determine the effect of simulated reverberation on speech perception in adults with normal hearing (Kreisman, 2003). This study used two reverberation simulations: a computer simulation utilizing the CATT-Acoustic software, and a hardware-generated simulation utilizing the Lexicon MPX-550 Effects Processor. Reverberation was simulated via both software and hardware simulations because it is not known which procedure may more closely approximate speech perception in actual rooms. Preliminary data has indicated that the computer simulation approximated the actual room reverberation (and subsequent speech-perception scores) more closely than the hardware simulation. Hopefully, such data will lead to the development of clinical procedures to assess speech perception in reverberation in the near future.

MEASURING REVERBERATION TIME WITH HARDWARE/SOFTWARE

Reverberation is often measured by presenting a high-intensity broad-band stimulus, such as white or pink noise, into an unoccupied room and measuring the amount of time required for that signal to decay 60 dB at various frequencies (Nabelek & Nabelek, 1994; Siebein, Crandell, & Gold, 1997). These measurements can be made in numerous ways. For example, various devices are commercially available, from highly technical computer-based devices that measure and record numerous aspects of the decay properties of an environment in great detail, to inexpensive, compact, battery-powered units that allow the audiologist to do simple measurements of RT. Audiologists frequently compute the average RT of a room by calculating the reverberation times at 500, 1,000, and 2,000 Hz. Average RT does not completely describe the RT of a room. For example, two very different rooms may have the same average RT. Specifically, one room may have predominantly low-frequency reverberation, while another room may have predominantly high-frequency reverberation. While both rooms have the same average RT, they may affect communication very differently. Therefore, when considering the impact of RT on speech perception, measuring and reporting RT as a function of frequency (e.g., for one-third-octave bands) is more helpful in order to describe more accurately the reverberation characteristics of the room.

MEASURING REVERBERATION TIME WITH FORMULAE

Reverberation also can be estimated via different formulae. Reverberation time was described by Sabine (1964) with the following formula:

$$RT_{60} = .161 \, V/Sa, \qquad (6.2)$$

where .161 is a constant, V is the volume of the room in cubic meters (0.049 if measuring in feet), and SSa is the total absorption of surfaces in the room. Sabine's formula assumes that the room has relatively normal proportions and that the reverberant sound field is diffuse. For smaller rooms, such as classrooms, Sabine's formula typically underestimates RT (Kosten, 1960; Siebein, Crandell, & Gold, 1997). Another formula that may be more appropriate for smaller rooms was developed by Fitzroy (1959):

$$RT_{60} = (0.049V/S^2) \, [(2(XY)/\,\alpha_{xy}) + (2(XZ)/\,\alpha_{xy}) + (2(XZ)/\,\alpha_{xy})], \qquad (6.3)$$

where V = volume of room in cubic feet, S = surface area of the room in square feet, X = room length, Y = room width, α = absorption coefficient, and Z = room height. Fitzroy's equation is based on calculations for the three main axes of reflections (floor to ceiling, side wall to side wall, and end wall to side wall).

Another equation for estimating RT in smaller rooms is the Norris-Eyring equation:

$$L_p = L_w + 10 \log \, [(Q/4\pi D^2) + (4/R)] + 10, \qquad (6.4)$$

where L_p = sound pressure level in decibels; L_w = sound power level in watts; Q = directivity of the sound source (1 = omnidirectional, 2 = hemispherical); D = distance from the sound source to the receiver; and R = room constant in Sabins of absorption (SSa). The Norris-Eyring formula is based on an average absorption coefficient for highly absorptive rooms (Siebein, Crandell, & Gold, 1997). The reader is referred to Egan (1987) for detailed examples of reverberation time using the aforementioned formulae.

USING A SIMPLIFIED PROCEDURE
TO ESTIMATE REVERBERATION TIME

A simple procedure for estimating RT in a classroom (Crandell, Smaldino, & Flexer, 1995) can be used to determine if more detailed measurements are worthwhile. A classroom acoustics documentation form is found in Appendix 6-A. The equipment needed for this procedure is a twenty-five-foot measuring tape (or ultrasonic distance estimator) and a calculator. The formula used for estimating classroom RT is RT =.05 V/A, where RT = reverberation time in seconds, .05 = a constant, V = volume of the room, and A = the total absorption of the room surfaces in Sabins. Note that all of the reverberation estimates will be conducted in unoccupied classrooms. Because a formula is used for this procedure, no improvement in measurement accuracy is obtained with teacher and students present. However, during more detailed measurements, the presence of room occupants would be desirable.

Step 1. Calculate the volume of the classroom. Volume is calculated by measuring the length, the width, and the height of the classroom in feet and multiplying them together (volume = length of room × width of room × height of room).

Step 2. Multiply the volume of the room by the constant .05 to obtain the numerator for the RT = 0.5 V/A equation.

Step 3. Determine the denominator of the equation. To do so, first measure the areas of the walls, ceiling, and floor of the room in square feet. If the walls, ceiling, or floor are irregularly shaped, measure each section separately. The area of the floor and ceiling is calculated by multiplying the length of the floor or ceiling by its width. The area of the walls can be determined by multiplying the length of each wall by its height.

Step 4. Determine the absorption coefficient (α) for the material composing the walls, ceiling, and floor. The absorption coefficient refers to a ratio of unreflected energy to incident energy present in a room; in other words, α is a measure of the sound reflectiveness of different construction materials. The coefficient is expressed in units called Sabins. Average absorption coefficients (at 500, 1,000, and 2,000 Hz) for the most common construction materials are presented in Table 6-1.

Step 5. Multiply the area of each floor, ceiling, and wall times the α of the material composing the surface. Add up all of the resultants of the multiplications to obtain the A in the denominator of the RT =.05 V/A equation. Recall that A = the total absorption of the room in Sabins.

Step 6. Calculate the estimated RT in seconds (RT = 0.5 V/A) by taking the numerator from Step 3 (.05 × V) and dividing it by the denominator from Step 6 (A = total absorption of the room in Sabins). If the RT is higher than 0.4 second, or if excessively high- or low-frequency reverberation is suspected, a more complete evaluation of reverberation should be conducted.

NOISE (SOUND-LEVEL) MEASUREMENTS IN THE CLASSROOM

All classrooms have the presence of some degree of background noise. Noise refers to the introduction of any undesired sound, or acoustic disturbance, in the classroom that can interfere with the perception of speech or other sounds

TABLE 6-1   Sound absorption coefficients for common materials found in classroom construction

Ceilings	Absorption Coefficient
Plaster, gypsum, lime on lathe	0.05
Suspended 5/8-inch acoustical tiles	0.68
Suspended 1/2-inch acoustical tiles	0.66
Not suspended 1/2-inch acoustical tiles	0.67
Suspended high absorptive panels	0.91

Floors	Absorption Coefficient
Linoleum	0.03
Wood parquet on concrete	0.06
Carpet on concrete	0.37
Carpet on foam padding	0.63

Walls	Absorption Coefficient
Brick	0.04
Painted concrete	0.07
Window glass	0.12
Plaster on concrete	0.12
Plywood	0.32
Concrete block	0.33

Source: Adapted from Berg (1993).

that a listener wants to hear (Finitzo-Hieber, 1988; Siebein, Crandell, & Gold, 1997). Noise may be generated from a variety of sources outside and inside the classroom. For example, traffic noise originates outside of the school building, and heating, ventilation, and air conditioning (HVAC) noise may originate outside or inside the school. Noise from the hallway and adjacent classrooms also may be present. In addition to these sources of noise, background noise can originate from within the room itself. Sources of noise in the room include children talking, chairs dragging on the floor, and the hum of fluorescent light fixtures, fans, and forced-air vents. Table 6-2 lists examples of external and internal noises.

The deleterious effects of noise on speech perception are well documented. Noise can degrade the perception of speech by distorting, or eliminating, the redundant acoustic and linguistic cues available in the signal (Cooper & Cutts, 1971; French & Steinberg, 1947; Miller, 1974; Miller & Nicely, 1955; Suter, 1978; Crandell, 1991a, 1991b; Moore, 1991; Danaher & Pickett, 1974). The spectral energy of consonant phonemes is less intense

TABLE 6-2 Common noise sources outside and inside the classroom

Outside School	Inside School	Inside Classroom
HVAC systems	Adjacent rooms	Students
Construction/ remodeling	Adjacent hallways	Chairs (dragging on floor)
Roadways	Adjacent HVAC systems	Desks (dragging on floor)
Trains	Construction/remodeling	Fluorescent light fixtures
Airplanes	Gymnasium	Computers
Playground	Cafeteria	Overhead projectors

than the energy of vowels; therefore, noise primarily affects the perception of consonant phonemes, making them less intelligible to the listener. Because as much as 90% of a listener's speech-perception ability is generated from consonant energy, this reduction of consonant perception can negatively influence speech perception.

The effectiveness of any given noise to reduce or eliminate (mask) speech cues depends on a number of parameters: (1) the long-term spectrum of the noise, (2) the intensity of the noise relative to the intensity of speech, and (3) the intensity fluctuations of the noise over time (Nabelek & Nabelek, 1994). Generally, low-frequency noises in a classroom environment are more effective maskers of speech than high-frequency noises because of upward spread of masking (Danaher & Pickett, 1974). The fact that low-frequency noises have a greater effect on speech perception than high-frequency noises is important because the spectra of noise found in classroom environments is predominantly low-frequency. The most effective masking noises appear to be those with spectra similar to the speech spectrum, as they affect all speech frequencies to the same degree.

MEASURING NOISE USING A SOUND-LEVEL METER

A sound-level meter, a device that measures the amplitude of sound, is one of the basic tools used to measure classroom acoustics. Sound-level meters range from small, inexpensive units that are battery powered to computer-based instruments that measure and record numerous properties of a signal. Sound-level meters are classified according to the ANSI S1.4 (American National Standards Institute, 1997) standards:

- Type I sound-level meters meet the most rigorous standards.
- Type II sound-level meters are for general use.
- Type III sound-level meters are for hobby use.

Sound-level meters often are used to determine the level of background noise. Background noise refers to any auditory disturbance within the room that interferes with what the listener wants to hear (Crandell, Smaldino, & Flexer, 1995). Such noise can originate from sources outside of the building, inside of the building, or inside the classroom. Measurement of room noise preferably is made with a Type I sound-level meter, although if this is unavailable, a Type II instrument could be used. Most sound-level meters incorporate weighting filter networks. These weighting scales, shown in Figure 6-1, are discussed below:

- The A-weighting network, or A-scale, is designed to simulate the sensitivity of the average human ear under conditions of moderate sound loudness (40 phons).
- The B-weighting network, or B-scale, is designed to simulate loud sound (70 phons).
- The C-weighting network, or C-scale, is designed to approximate how the ear would respond to very loud sound.

The A-weighting network is conventionally used for room and factory noise measurements. However, it is critical to understand that a single number obtained from the sound pressure measurement can be obtained from a number of very different spectra.

A spectral analysis of the classroom signal and noise would provide a more accurate measurement of the spectral intensity within a classroom. Spectral

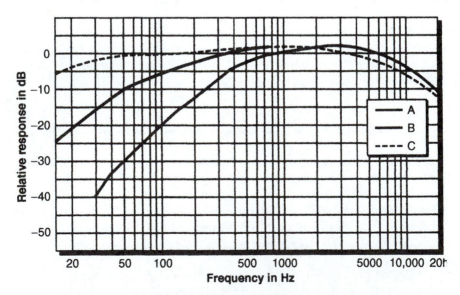

Figure 6-1. Weighting scales for sound-level meters.

analysis is usually made from 63 to 8,000 Hz. Such analysis requires an octave-band filter network for the sound-level meter. If such equipment is available, Noise Criteria Curves (NCCs) can be established to determine the effects of noise on speech perception within the classroom (Beranek, 1954). NCCs are a family of frequency-intensity curves based on octave-band sound pressure across a 20–10,000 Hz band and have been related to successful use of an acoustic space for a variety of activities (Figure 6-2). The value of each NCC is determined by finding the highest NCC the sound pressure intersects. Generally, the NCC rating is 8 to 10 dB below the dBA level of that room. Therefore, whenever possible it is recommended that background noise levels in classrooms be measured via NCC measures, as this procedure gives the examiner additional information regarding the spectral characteristics of the noise.

With this information, the audiologist or acoustical engineer can isolate and modify sources of excessive noise in the classroom. Table 6-3 presents appropriate NCC values and related A-weighted values. The effects of different NCC values on communicative efficiency are shown in Table 6-4. An NCC of 20–25 is considered suitable for a classroom. The equivalent A-weighted sound-pressure level would be approximately 30–35 dBA. Stated differently, 30–35 dBA would be the target sound-pressure level for the long-term average noise spectrum in a classroom. Room Criteria (RC) curves are a similar concept to NCCs. RC curves are designed to include frequencies commonly associated with mechanical noises such as heating, ventilation, and air conditioning

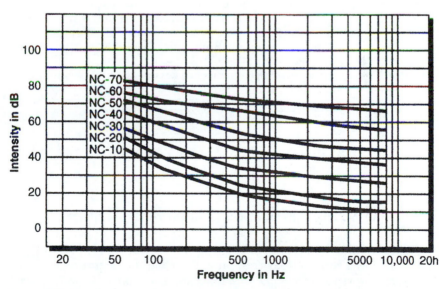

Figure 6-2. Noise Criteria Curves for an average occupied classroom setting and conversational speech.

TABLE 6-3 Appropriate NCC values, and related A-weighting values, for various communication environments

Listening Space	NC Curve	Equivalent dBA Levels
Broadcast studios	15–20	25–30
Concert halls	15–20	25–30
Classrooms (no amplification)	25	35
Apartments and hotels	25–30	30–35
Homes (sleeping areas)	25–35	35–45
Libraries	30	40–45
Restaurants	45	55

Source: Adapted from Berg (1993).

TABLE 6-4 The effects of different NCC values on communicative efficacy

NC Curve	Communication Environment
20–30	Very quiet office, telephone use satisfactory, suitable for large conferences
30–35	Quiet office, satisfactory for conferences at 15-foot table, normal voice at 10–30 feet, telephone use satisfactory
35–40	Satisfactory for conferences at 6–8-foot table, telephone use satisfactory, normal voice at 6–12 feet
40–50	Satisfactory for conferences at 4–5-foot table, telephone use may be difficult, normal voice at 3–6 feet, raised voice to 12 feet
50–55	Unsatisfactory for conferences of more than two to three people, telephone use can be difficult, normal voice at 1–2 feet, raised voice at 3–6 feet
More than 55	Very noisy, office environment is unsatisfactory, telephone use is difficult

Source: Adapted from Berg (1993).

(HVAC) units. For this purpose, the NCCs were modified at very high and very low frequencies to produce RC curves.

A SIMPLIFIED PROCEDURE FOR ESTIMATING NOISE

Background noise in a classroom can be estimated using (1) a sound-level meter that has A-scale and slow response, (2) a 25-foot measuring tape, and (3) a standard reading passage. The following procedure (Crandell, Smaldino, & Flexer, 1995) can be used:

Step 1. Position the teacher in the most common instructional position in the classroom. The students should be seated in their normal seats for instruction. Acoustical measurements should be made in the time period when instruction normally occurs so that the conditions are representative of actual instructional environments.

Step 2. Turn on the sound-level meter. Set the sound-level meter on the A-scale or weighting and on slow response. If the meter allows the dB range to be defined, set it to accommodate 40–60 dB SPL to begin.

Step 3. Position the sound-level meter to approximate the center of each selected student's head while seated in the desk. Point the sound-level meter toward the teacher position. Be sure that your body is not in the sound path between teacher and student, as this will produce inaccurate measurements. At a minimum, student desks at the four corners, the middle, and the middle back of the classroom seating should be measured. More locations can be measured if desired.

Step 4. Measure the ambient noise level at the selected student locations with the students quiet, and record this level on the classroom documentation form. If the noise level fluctuates, take three measurements at one-minute intervals, average the readings, and record those on the form. These measurements will provide an estimate of the ambient noise level during an instructional period. If measurements can only be made when the classroom is unoccupied, you may convert the unoccupied noise levels to occupied by adding 10 dB to each unoccupied measurement. This conversion is roughly equal to the known difference in noise level between average occupied and unoccupied classrooms.

Step 5. The teacher should begin reading the standard reading passage at a normal instructional intensity level.

Step 6. Repeat Step 4, now that the teacher is reading the standard passage. These measurements provide an estimate of the signal level during an instructional period.

Step 7. Subtract the ambient noise measurement (obtained in Step 4) from the teacher voice measurement (obtained in Step 6) to determine the S/N ratio of the classroom at the selected student sites. For example, a student location with a teacher voice level of 60 dBA and a noise level of 50 dBA would have an S/N ratio of +10 dB. A student location with a teacher voice level of 60 dBA and a noise level of 70 dBA would have an S/N ratio of –10 dB.

CLASSROOM RECOMMENDATIONS

The following steps are suggested for developing acoustical recommendations for a classroom. Acoustical modifications are discussed in greater detail in the next chapter.

Step 1. Compare the classroom acoustic results to the classroom standards (discussed in Chapter 5). If the classroom meets or exceeds the standards, no acoustic modification is necessary. However, if the classroom does not meet the standards—and many classroom do not (Knecht, Nelson, Whitelaw, & Feth, 2002)—acoustic modification should be attempted alone or in addition to Steps 2–4.

Step 2. Inspect the classroom geometry on the classroom documentation form to determine if a reduction of distance between teacher and students is possible. Speaker-listener distance affects both S/N ratio and RT. Reducing the speaker-listener distance can be expected to increase the signal slightly as well as potentially increase speech perception due to increased early reflections.

Step 3. Adverse RT can be affected by structural changes within a classroom, such as adding acoustical ceiling tile or carpeting the floor. Structural changes have been described elsewhere (see Chapter 3) and will not be repeated here. It is important to note that structural changes are often cost-prohibitive and are not frequently used to improve classroom acoustics.

Step 4. Install a sound field FM amplification system in the classroom. An ideal sound field installation increases the teacher's voice approximately 10 dB.

Step 5. Given that you have intervened in ways described in Steps 1–4, determine whether the intervention accomplished the anticipated goal. As previously noted, the goal is to increase the level of the teacher's voice 10 dB uniformly throughout the classroom measurement locations.

Step 6. Repeat the teacher voice level measurements with the intervention in place and record the new voice levels. If these measurements are 10 dB or greater at each student location measured, the goal has been accomplished. If the levels do not attain the goal, modification or additional intervention is necessary.

SUMMARY

The environmental characteristics of most classrooms are continually fluctuating. Nevertheless, it is imperative to ascertain the function that a classroom serves throughout the day before measuring the acoustical environment and recommending possible improvements. The acoustical environment should be measured in terms of reverberation time and noise, as both of these factors have been demonstrated to affect speech perception. Reverberation time can be estimated via various formulae or can be measured using hardware or software devices. Techniques utilizing simulated reverberation are currently being examined to more conveniently assess the effects of reverberation time on speech perception. Noise is typically measured via a sound-level meter. The effects of noise on speech perception can further be determined by establishing NC and RC curves. Acoustical recommendations for a classroom may be formally developed following the outline provided in this chapter.

DISCUSSION TOPICS

1. Discuss different procedures for measuring noise in the classroom.
2. Discuss different procedures for measuring reverberation in the classroom.
3. Which formulae appear to be the most appropriate for measuring reverberation in a classroom? Discuss why.
4. What are advantages of measuring noise with NC curves compared to using an A-weighted scale?

REFERENCES

American National Standards Institute (1997). Specification for sound level meters. ANSI S1.4–1983 (R1997), New York, NY.

Beranek, L. (1954). *Acoustics.* New York: McGraw-Hill.

Berg, F. (1993). *Acoustics and sound systems in schools.* Clifton Park, NY: Thomson Delmar Learning.

Bolt, R., & MacDonald, A. (1949). Theory of speech masking by reverberation. *Journal of the Acoustical Society of America, 21,* 577–580.

Bradley, J. (1986). Speech intelligibility studies in classrooms. *Journal of the Acoustical Society of America, 80,* 846–854.

Cooper, J., & Cutts, B. (1971). Speech discrimination in noise. *Journal of Speech and Hearing Research, 14,* 332–337.

Crandell, C. (1991a). Classroom acoustics for normal hearing children: Implications for rehabilitation. *Educational Audiology Monograph, 2,* 18–38.

Crandell, C. (1991b). Individual differences in speech recognition ability: Implications for hearing aid selection. *Ear and Hearing, 12,* 100–108.

Crandell, C. (1992). Classroom acoustics for hearing-impaired children. *Journal of the Acoustical Society of America, 92,* 2470.

Crandell, C., & Bess, F. (1986). Speech recognition of children in a "typical" classroom setting. *American Speech, Language, & Hearing Association, 29,* 87.

Crandell., C., Smaldino, J., & Flexer, C. (1995). *Sound field FM amplification: Theory and practical applications.* San Diego: Singular Publishing Company.

Crum, D. (1974). The effects of noise, reverberation, and speaker-to-listener distance on speech understanding. Unpublished doctoral dissertation. Northwestern University, Evanston, IL.

Danaher, E., & Pickett, J. (1974). Some masking effects produced by low frequency vowel formants in persons with sensorineural hearing loss. *Journal of Speech and Hearing Research, 18,* 261–271.

Egan, M. (1987). *Architectural acoustics.* New York: McGraw-Hill Book Company.

Finitzo-Hieber, T. (1988). Classroom acoustics. In R. Roeser & M. Downs (Eds.), *Auditory Disorders in School Children* (2nd ed., pp. 221–233). New York: Thieme-Stratton.

Finitzo-Hieber, T., & Tillman, T. (1978). Room acoustics effects on monosyllabic word discrimination ability for normal and hearing-impaired children. *Journal of Speech and Hearing Research, 21,* 440–458.

Fitzroy, D. (1959). Reverberation formula that seems to be more accurate with non-uniform distribution of absorption. *Journal of the Acoustical Society of America, 31,* 893–897.

French, N., & Steinberg, J. (1947). Factors governing the intelligibility of speech sounds. *Journal of the Acoustical Society of America, 19,* 90–119.

Gelfand, S., & Silman, S. (1979). Effects of small room reverberation upon the recognition of some consonant features. *Journal of the Acoustical Society of America, 66,* 22–29.

Knecht, H. A., Nelson, P. B., Whitelaw, G. M., & Feth, L. L. (2002). Background noise levels and reverberation times in unoccupied classrooms: Predictions and measurements. *American Journal of Audiology, 11,* 65–71.

Knudsen, V., & Harris, C. (1978). *Acoustical designing in architecture.* New York: American Institute of Physics for the Acoustical Society of America.

Kosten, C. (1960). International comparison measurements in the reverberation room. *Acustica, 10,* 400–411.

Kreisman, B. (2003). Simulated reverberation and speech perception: Clinical implications. Paper presented at the American Academy of Audiology 15th Annual Convention, San Antonio, TX.

Kurtovic, H. (1975). The influence of reflected sound upon speech intelligibility. *Acustica, 33,* 32–39.

Lochner, J., & Burger, J. (1964). The influence of reflections in auditorium acoustics. *Journal of Sound & Vibration, 4,* 426–454.

Miller, G. (1974). Effects of noise on people. *Journal of the Acoustical Society of America, 56,* 724–764.

Miller, G., & Nicely, P. (1955). An analysis of perceptual confusions among some English consonants. *Journal of the Acoustical Society of America, 27,* 338–352.

Moore, B. (1991). *An introduction to the psychology of hearing.* New York: Academic Press.

Nabelek, A., & Nabelek, I. (1994). Room acoustics and speech perception. In J. Katz (Ed.), *Handbook of clinical audiology* (4th ed., pp. 624–637). Baltimore: Williams and Wilkins.

Nabelek, A., & Pickett, J. (1974a). Monaural and binaural speech perception through hearing aids under noise and reverberation with normal and hearing impaired listeners. *Journal of Speech & Hearing Research, 17,* 724–739.

Nabelek, A., & Pickett, J. (1974b). Reception of consonants in a classroom as affected by monaural and binaural listening, noise, reverberation, and hearing aids. *Journal of the Acoustical Society of America, 56,* 628–639.

Nabelek, A., & Robinette, L. (1978). Reverberation as a parameter in clinical testing. *Audiology, 17,* 239–259.

Sabine, W. (1964). *Collected papers on acoustics.* New York: Dover.

Siebein, G., Crandell, C., & Gold, M. (1997). Principles of classroom acoustics: Reverberation. *Educational Audiology Monograph, 5,* 32–43.

Suter, A. (1978). The ability of mildly hearing impaired individuals to discriminate speech in noise. Aerospace Medical Research Laboratory Report No. AMRL-RT-78–4. Wright Patterson Air Force Base, Ohio.

APPENDIX 6-A
CLASSROOM ACOUSTICS DOCUMENTATION FORM

Classroom Acoustics Documentation Form

Date _____

Teacher_____ Grade _____

Audiologist_____

FM SFA System Used _____

CLASSROOM SCHEMATIC DIAGRAM

	Nearest		Farthest	
TEACHER-LISTENER DISTANCE:	_____feet		_____feet

TEACHER VOICE LEVEL IN dBA:

Unamplified			*Amplified*
Location A	_____	Location A	_____
Location B	_____	Location B	_____
Location C	_____	Location C	_____
Location D	_____	Location D	_____
Location E	_____	Location E	_____
Location F	_____	Location F	_____
Location G	_____	Location G	_____

REVERBERATION TIME

Room Volume (V) = _____cubic feet

Area Floor	_____X Abs. Coef. _____ = A Floor	_____
Area Ceiling	_____X Abs. Coef. _____ = A Ceiling	_____
Area Side Wall 1	_____X Abs. Coef. _____ = A Wall 1	_____
Area Side Wall 2	_____X Abs. Coef. _____ = A Wall 2	_____
Area End Wall 1	_____X Abs. Coef. _____ = A End 1	_____
Area End Wall 2	_____X Abs. Coef. _____ = A End 2	_____
		Total A _____

RT of classroom = .05 X _____(V) / _____(A) = _____seconds

CHAPTER 7

Acoustical Modifications in Classrooms

Carl C. Crandell, PhD
Joseph J. Smaldino, PhD

KEY POINTS

- In 2002, *ANSI S12.60–2002: Acoustical Performance Criteria, Design Requirements, and Guidelines for Schools* was officially published.
- The basic provisions of the standard are Reverberation Times = 0.6 second small rooms/0.7 second large rooms; Background Sound Level = 35 dBA.
- Ambient classroom noise can originate from external noise (noise that is generated from outside the school); internal noise (noise that originates from within the school building, but outside the classroom); and classroom noise (noise that is generated within the classroom).
- Noise sources must be isolated and treated prior to the installation of any amplification technology.

The speech-recognition difficulties experienced by children with hearing impairment and children with normal hearing highlight the need to provide an appropriate listening environment for these populations. Recall from previous chapters that acoustical guidelines and standards for such populations indicate that signal-to-noise (S/N) ratios should exceed +15 dB; unoccupied noise levels should not exceed 30–35 dB(A), while reverberation times should not surpass 0.4 second. As previously noted, however, these acoustical recommendations are rarely achieved in real-world listening environments. This chapter will examine various modifications of the acoustical environment to facilitate the speech perception of pediatric listeners in educational environments. For additional discussions pertaining to acoustical modifications in the classroom, the reader is directed to Beranek (1954), Bess and McConnell (1981), Crandell (1992), Crandell and Smaldino (1995a, 1995b), Finitzo-Hieber (1988), Finitzo-Hieber and Tillman (1978), Knudsen and Harris (1978), Niemoller (1968), Olsen (1977, 1981, 1988), and Ross (1978). This chapter also provides a brief overview of ANSI S12.60–2002.

ANSI S12.60–2002: ACOUSTICAL PERFORMANCE CRITERIA, DESIGN REQUIREMENTS, AND GUIDELINES FOR SCHOOLS

In 2002 (ANSI, 2002), this landmark standard was published. Compliance with the specifications of the standard is currently voluntary, but it is hoped that in the future good classroom acoustics will be considered as a universal design element and built into every classroom. The objectives of the standard were to develop acoustic criteria that would produce an adequate environment for listening and learning in the classroom as well as improve acoustic privacy between rooms. In order to meet these objectives, performance criteria specifications for allowable background noise and reverberation and design guidelines for attenuating noise entering learning spaces were developed. The basic provisions of the standard are as follows:

RT60-Reverberation Time
- 0.6 second small rooms
- 0.7 second large rooms

Background Sound Level
- 35 dBA
- Assume 50 dB teacher level: +15 SNR

Partition Design
- Between classrooms: 50 STC
- Between corridor and classroom: 45 STC
- Between high noise room and classroom: 60 STC

REDUCTION OF NOISE AND REVERBERATION LEVELS IN THE CLASSROOM

Recall that ambient classroom noise can originate from several possible sources. These sources include external noise (noise that is generated from outside the school); internal noise (noise that originates from within the school building but outside the classroom); and classroom noise (noise that is generated within the classroom). In order to conduct the most appropriate modification of the classroom, the first determination is which specific noise source, or sources, needs to be reduced. Moreover, the reverberant characteristics of the enclosure must be quantified. With these considerations in mind, the remainder of this chapter will outline various procedures in order to reduce noise and reverberation levels in the classroom. Acoustical modification of the classroom must be conducted prior to sound field utilization.

Reduction of External Noise Levels

- Rooms utilized for the hearing impaired, or for normal hearers, must be located away from high noise sources, such as busy automobile traffic, railroads, construction sites, airports, and furnace/air conditioning units. The most effective procedure for achieving this goal is through appropriate planning with contractors, school officials, architects, architectural engineers, audiologists, and teachers for the hearing impaired before the design and construction of the school building. Such consultation should include strategies for locating rooms away from high external noise sources. Moreover, acoustical modifications such as the placement of vibration-reduction pads underneath the supporting beams of the building to reduce structure-borne sounds can be implemented. Unfortunately, acoustic planning prior to building construction is rare (Crandell & Smaldino, 1992, 1995a, 1995b; Crandell, Smaldino, & Flexer, 1995).

- A Sound Transmission Loss (STL) of at least 45 to 50 dB is often required for external walls. Sound Transmission Loss refers to the amount of noise that is attenuated as it passes through a material. If an external noise of 100 dB SPL was reduced to 60 dB SPL in the room, the exterior wall of that room would have an STL of 40 dB SPL. A seven-inch concrete wall provides approximately 53 dB attenuation of outside noise, while windows and doors provide only 24 dB and 20 dB attenuation, respectively. Therefore, doors and windows on the external wall should be avoided in situations of high external noise levels. Average STL values for different structures can be found in most books published on acoustics. Procedures to increase the STL of an external wall include (1) the placement of absorptive materials, such as fiberglass, between the wall studs; (2) thick or double concrete construction on the exterior wall; and (3) the addition of several layers of gypsum board or plywood material.

- All exterior walls must be free of cracks or openings that would allow extraneous noises into the room. Even small openings in external walls can significantly reduce the STL.

- If windows are located on the external wall, they must be properly installed, heavy-weighted or double-paned (such as storm windows), and should remain closed (whenever possible) if high external noise sources exist. In addition, existing windows can be sealed with non-hardening caulk to increase the STL. Of course, safety regulations must be checked before sealing outside windows.
- Landscaping strategies can also attenuate external noise sources. These strategies include the placement of nondeciduous trees or shrubs and earthen banks around the school building.
- Solid concrete barriers with an STL of 30–35 dB can be placed between the school building and the noise source to reduce external noise entering into the room.

Reduction of Internal Noise Levels

- Often, the most cost-effective procedure for reducing internal noise levels in the room is to relocate the children in that room to a quieter area of the building. Rooms used for communication must not be located next to a high noise source such as the gymnasium, metal shop, cafeteria, or band room. At least one quiet environment, such as a storage area or closet, should separate rooms from each other or from high noise sources in the school building.
- If suspended ceilings separate the room from another room, then sound-absorbing materials should be placed in the plenum space above the wall.
- Double- or thick-wall construction should be used for the interior walls, particularly those walls that face noisy hallways or rooms. Additional layers of gypsum board or plywood, or the placement of absorptive materials between wall studding, can also increase the attenuation characteristics of interior wall surfaces. Moreover, all cracks between rooms should be sealed.
- Acoustical ceiling tile and/or carpeting can be used in hallways outside the room.
- All rooms should contain acoustically treated or well-fitting high mass per unit area doors (preferably with rubber or gasket seals). Hollow-core doors between rooms and facing the hallway should not be utilized. Doors (or interior walls) should not contain ventilation ducts that lead into the hallways.
- Heating or cooling ducts that serve more than one room can be lined with acoustical materials or furnished with baffles to decrease noise emitting from one room to another.
- Permanently mounted blackboards can be backed with absorptive materials to reduce sound transmission from adjacent rooms.

Reduction of Room Noise Levels

- The simplest procedure to reduce the effects of room noise is to position children away from high noise sources such as fans, air conditioners, or heating ducts; faulty lighting fixtures; and doors or windows adjacent to sources of noise. Often, however, room noise sources are so intense that no location in the room is appropriate for communication. In these cases, acoustical modification of the room must be conducted.

- Malfunctioning air conduction or heating units and ducts should be replaced or acoustically treated. Heating ducts, for example, can be lined with acoustical materials or fit with silencers to reduce both vibratory and airborne noise. In addition, rubber supports and flexible sleeves or joints should be used to reduce the transmission of structural-borne noise through the ductwork. Moreover, all fans and electrical motors in air conditioning and heating units must be lubricated and maintained on a regular basis.

- Installation of thick wall-to-wall carpeting (with adequate padding) to dampen the noise of shuffling of hard-soled shoes, the movement of desks and chairs, etc., can reduce room noise levels.

- Acoustical paneling can be placed on the walls and ceiling. Wall paneling typically should be placed partly down the wall and not on walls parallel to one another.

- The placement of some form of rubber tips on the legs of desks and chairs can decrease room noise. This recommendation is particularly important if the room is not carpeted.

- Acoustically treated furniture can be purchased for rooms. It must be noted that such furniture can be expensive and may present hygiene problems.

- Hanging of thick curtains or acoustically treated venetian blinds over window areas to dampen room noise levels can be effective.

- Avoid open-plan rooms for children, as such rooms are considerably noisier than regular rooms.

- Instruction should not take place in areas separated from other teaching areas by sliding doors, thin partitions, or temporary walls. Walls between instruction areas must be of sufficient thickness and continuous between the solid ceiling and floor. Walls that are not continuous allow for significant sound transmission between rooms.

- Fluorescent lighting systems, including the ballast, need to be regularly maintained and replaced if faulty.

- Typewriter or computer keyboard noise can be lowered by the placement of rubber pads, or carpet remnants, under such instruments. Whenever possible, such instruments (as well as any other office equipment) should be located in separate rooms. Rubber pads to reduce vibratory noise should be placed under all office equipment in the school.

- Children can be encouraged to wear soft-soled shoes.

Reduction of Room Reverberation

The presence, or absence, of absorptive surfaces within a room will affect the reverberant characteristics of that environment. Materials with hard, smooth surfaces such as concrete, cinder block, and hard plaster are poor absorbers, while materials with soft, rough-surfaced, or porous surfaces (cloth, fiberglass, corkboard) tend to be good absorbers of sound. Hence, rooms with bare cement walls, floors, or ceilings tend to exhibit higher RTs than rooms that contain absorptive surfaces such as carpeting, draperies, and acoustical ceiling tile. A useful index in determining the reverberant characteristics of a room is the absorption coefficient. Absorption coefficient (α) refers to the ratio of unreflected energy to incident energy present in a room. A surface with an absorption coefficient of 1.00 would technically absorb 100% of all reflections, while a surface structure with an absorption coefficient of 0.00 would reflect all of the incident sound. Table 7-1 provides a summary of absorption coefficients for different materials. Note that the absorption coefficients, which are typically indicated from 125 to 4,000 Hz, are frequency dependent.

Specifically, most surface materials in a room do not absorb low-frequency sounds as effectively as high-frequency sounds. Due to these absorption characteristics, room reverberation is often shorter at higher frequencies than in lower-frequency regions. Generally, surfaces are not considered absorptive until they reach an absorption coefficient of 0.20. There may be a tendency when excessive reverberation occurs to treat most or all of the surfaces in a room with sound-absorbing materials. If all of the surfaces become sound absorbent, then the teacher is effectively speaking in an anechoic or non-reverberant environment and will have to raise her or his voice or use an amplification system to overcome the lack of reflected sounds that would normally be present in a room. The next section discusses several procedures to reduce reverberation in a room.

Procedures to Reduce Room Reverberation

- Reverberation can be reduced by covering the hard reflective surfaces in a room with absorptive materials such as acoustical paneling. To reduce reverberation, ceilings should be covered with acoustical paneling. The ceiling should contain an acoustical tile ceiling. The acoustical tile should be suspended from the structural deck and have an absorption coefficient of at least 0.65. This will absorb multiple-order sound reflections from the corners of the room and reduce the RT to acceptable levels. Acoustical panels may also be placed on walls but typically not on walls parallel to one another. Cork bulletin boards, carpeting, and bookcases can also be strategically placed on the walls; however, such materials are not as absorptive as acoustical paneling. Interestingly, the installation of absorptive materials will not only reduce reverberation in the environment, but also will decrease the noise level in the room by 5–8 dB.

TABLE 7-1   Sound absorption coefficient for various types of acoustical treatments and for building materials

Material	Frequency (Hz)					
	125	250	500	1k	2k	4k
Walls						
Brick	0.03	0.03	0.03	0.04	0.05	0.07
Concrete painted	0.10	0.05	0.06	0.07	0.09	0.08
Window glass	0.35	0.25	0.18	0.12	0.07	0.04
Marble	0.01	0.01	0.01	0.02	0.02	0.00
Plaster or concrete	0.12	0.09	0.07	0.05	0.05	0.04
Plywood	0.28	0.22	0.17	0.09	0.10	0.11
Concrete block, coarse	0.36	0.44	0.31	0.29	0.39	0.25
Heavyweight drapery	0.14	0.35	0.55	0.72	0.70	0.65
Fiberglass wall treatment, 1 inch (2.5 cm)	0.08	0.32	0.99	0.76	0.34	0.12
Fiberglass wall treatment, 7 inch (17.8 cm)	0.86	0.99	0.99	0.99	0.99	0.99
Wood paneling on glass fiber blanket	0.40	0.99	0.80	0.50	0.40	0.30
Floors						
Wood parquet on concrete	0.04	0.04	0.07	0.60	0.06	0.07
Linoleum	0.02	0.03	0.03	0.03	0.03	0.02
Carpet on concrete	0.02	0.06	0.14	0.37	0.60	0.65
Carpet on foam rubber padding	0.08	0.24	0.57	0.69	0.71	0.73
Ceilings						
Plaster, gypsum, or line on lath	0.14	0.10	0.06	0.05	0.04	0.03
Acoustic tiles ⅝ inch (1.6 cm), suspended 16 inches (40.6 cm) from ceiling	0.25	0.28	0.46	0.71	0.86	0.93
Acoustic tiles 1/2 inch (1.2 cm), suspended 16 inches (40.6 cm) from ceiling	0.52	0.37	0.50	0.69	0.79	0.78
The same as above, but cemented directly to ceiling	0.10	0.22	0.61	0.56	0.74	0.72
High absorptive panels, 1 inch (2.5 cm), suspended 16 inches (40.6 cm) from ceiling	0.58	0.88	0.75	0.99	1.00	0.96

(continued)

TABLE 7-1 *(continued)*

Material	Frequency (Hz)					
	125	250	500	1k	2k	4k
Upholstered seats	0.19	0.37	0.56	0.67	0.61	0.59
Audience in upholstered seats	0.39	0.57	0.80	0.94	0.92	0.87
Grass	0.11	0.26	0.60	0.69	0.92	0.99
Soil	0.15	0.25	0.40	0.55	0.60	0.60
Water surface	0.01	0.01	0.01	0.02	0.02	0.03

Source: Adapted from Lipscomb (1978).

- Thick carpeting on the floors can also significantly reduce reverberation and noise in a room. Rooms that contain both ceiling tile and carpets have approximately 60% of room surfaces covered with absorptive material. However, rooms with just the ceiling and floor covered are prone to acoustical defects such as flutter echoes. Flutter echoes are the continued reflection of sound waves between two opposite parallel surfaces. This is a particular problem in small rooms such as classrooms. It can be heard as a distinctive slapping or ringing sound. Absorbing materials can be placed on the walls, or the walls can be splayed slightly to reduce this problem. Sound absorbent acoustical panels (one-inch thick minimum) can be placed on the sidewalls at the front of the room to reduce flutter in the area where the teacher speaks.
- Curtains or thick draperies can be placed to cover the hard reflective surfaces of windows. Even when the curtains are open, they will serve to minimally reduce the RT of the enclosure.
- Positioning of mobile bulletin boards and blackboards at angles other than parallel to opposite walls will also reduce the reflected sound in an enclosure.
- Some teachers have used creative artwork from egg cartons or carpet scraps attached to walls or suspended from ceilings to help absorb noise and reduce reverberation. Safety regulations must be checked before placing in the room materials that may not be fire-retardant.
- Recall that as room size increases, so does RT. Therefore, keeping classrooms small and designing rooms with moderate ceiling heights is an important consideration. A ceiling height of approximately ten to thirteen feet is usually acceptable.
- In rooms where greater teacher-to-student distances are encountered, such as middle schools and high schools, it is useful to provide a surface to reflect sound waves to the students. This becomes relatively easy in rooms that are used for conventional lecture-style teaching. An area of the room can be designated as the teaching area. This is the location from which the teacher will speak. The acoustical design issue is to

provide early sound reflections from the ceiling to seats in the room. The front part of the ceiling should be gypsum board, plaster, or other sound-reflecting material. This will allow early sound reflections from the teacher's voice to reinforce the direct sound and increase the loudness of sound reaching students in the room.

- Curtains or thick draperies can be placed to cover the hard reflective surfaces of windows. However, curtains can be a maintenance problem for the school.

CURRENT STATUS OF ACOUSTICAL MODIFICATIONS IN CLASSROOMS

Despite the numerous procedures for treating the acoustical environment, classrooms often exhibit minimal degrees of acoustical modifications. Bess, Sinclair, and Riggs (1984) reported that while 100% of classrooms had acoustical ceiling tile, only 68% had carpeting, and only 13% had draperies. None of the classrooms contained any form of acoustical furniture treatment. Crandell and Smaldino (1995b) reported that while all of thirty-two classrooms examined had acoustic ceiling tile, only fourteen (54%) contained carpeting. Moreover, only one of the classrooms had drapes, while none of the rooms had acoustical furniture treatments.

SUMMARY

While compliance with the provisions of the new ANSI standard for classroom acoustics is voluntary, improving classroom acoustic conditions is the right thing to do. This chapter overviews some of the practical ways in which background noise and reverberation can be reduced. Implementation of these reduction methods in conjunction with amplification technology can significantly improve the classroom acoustic environment for listening and learning.

DISCUSSION TOPICS

1. How can structural sound be reduced?
2. What is sound transmission loss? What do typical external walls require for sound transmission loss?
3. What are three ways to reduce external noise?
4. What are three ways that internal noise can be reduced?
5. What are three ways that classroom noise can be reduced?

6. What are good absorbers of sound? What would an absorption coefficient of 0.00 do? When are surfaces considered absorptive?

7. What would happen if the whole room became sound absorbent?

REFERENCES

ANSI (2002). *ANSI S12.60, Acoustical performance criteria, design requirements, and guidelines for schools.* New York: American National Standards Institute.

Beranek, L. (1954). *Acoustics.* New York: McGraw-Hill.

Bess, F., & McConnell, F. (1981). *Audiology, education and the hearing-impaired child.* St. Louis: C. V. Mosby.

Bess, F., Sinclair, J., & Riggs, D. (1984). Group amplification in schools for the hearing-impaired. *Ear and Hearing, 5,* 138–144.

Crandell, C. (1992). Classroom acoustics for hearing-impaired children. *Journal of the Acoustical Society of America, 92*(4), 2470.

Crandell, C., & Smaldino, J. (1995a). The importance of room acoustics. In R. Tyler & D. Schum (Eds.), *Assistive listening devices* (pp. 142–164). Baltimore: Allyn & Bacon.

Crandell, C., & Smaldino, J. (1995b). An update of classroom acoustics for children with hearing impairment. *Volta Review, 6,* 18–25.

Crandell, C., Smaldino, J., & Flexer, C. (1995). *Sound-field FM amplification: Theory and practical applications.* Clifton Park, NY: Thomson Delmar Learning.

Finitzo-Hieber, T. (1988). Classroom acoustics. In R. Roeser & M. Downs (Eds.), *Auditory disorders in school children* (2nd ed., pp. 221–233). New York: Thieme-Stratton.

Finitzo-Hieber, T., & Tillman, T. (1978). Room acoustics effects on monosyllabic word discrimination ability for normal and hearing-impaired children. *Journal of Speech and Hearing Research, 21,* 440–458.

Knudsen, V., & Harris, C. (1978). *Acoustical designing in architecture.* Washington, DC: The American Institute of Physics for the Acoustical Society of America.

Lipscomb, D. (1978). *Noise in audiology.* Austin, TX: Pro-Ed.

Niemoller, A. (1968). Acoustical design of classrooms for the deaf. *American Annals of the Deaf, 113,* 1040–1045.

Olsen, W. (1977). Acoustics and amplification in classrooms for the hearing impaired. In F. H. Bess (Ed.), *Childhood deafness: Causation, assessment and management.* New York: Grune & Stratton.

Olsen, W. (1981). The effects of noise and reverberation on speech intelligibility. In F. H. Bess, B. A. Freeman, & J. S. Sinclair (Eds.), *Amplification in education.* Washington, DC: Alexander Graham Bell Association for the Deaf.

Olsen, W. (1988). Classroom acoustics for hearing-impaired children. In F. H. Bess (Ed.), *Hearing impairment in children.* Parkton, MD: York Press.

Ross, M. (1978). Classroom acoustics and speech intelligibility. In J. Katz (Ed.), *Handbook of clinical audiology.* Baltimore: Williams & Wilkins.

CHAPTER 8

Sound Field Amplification: Steps to Placement in the Classroom

Joseph J. Smaldino, PhD
Carl C. Crandell, PhD
Carol Flexer, PhD

KEY POINTS

- There are distinct advantages and disadvantages to using sound field amplification. Both should be considered when deciding the best way to deal with less than desirable room acoustics.
- Adequate sound levels and distribution of spoken instruction in a classroom can be accomplished by using either a pragmatic or simulation approach to installation.
- Infrared sound field systems have certain advantages over FM-based systems—and some disadvantages.
- Sound field systems can be used with other technologies designed for children who are deaf or hard of hearing, so compatibility must be considered.

Previous chapters have demonstrated that speech perception and academic performance can be severely compromised by inappropriate classroom acoustics. The primary acoustical considerations are classroom noise level, signal-to-noise (S/N) ratio, reverberation time (RT), and distance from the teacher. Due to the adverse effects of these variables on pyschoeducational performance, classroom acoustical modifications and sound field amplification must be considered as a universal design element in educational settings. Like adequate lighting in the room, a student's access to a high-quality speech signal must occur in classrooms for appropriate education to occur. With these considerations in mind, this chapter will examine practical applications for the placement of sound field amplification in the classroom. Specifically, this chapter will identify and discuss issues important in considering the selection, installation, and use of sound field amplification systems, including (1) wireless microphone modality, (2) cost factors, (3) appropriate FM carrier frequencies, (4) evaluating the number of available discrete channels used by various manufacturers, (5) compatibility of systems, (6) number and positioning of loudspeakers, (7) durability, flexibility, portability, and ease of installation of the sound field amplification equipment, (8) fidelity of equipment, (9) where to position children with a known hearing impairment or perceptual deficit in an amplified classroom, (10) microphone style, (11) inservice training and follow-up issues, (12) combined sound field and personal FM use, and (13) feedback control. Prior to this discussion, however, the reader is directed to Tables 8-1 and 8-2 for advantages and disadvantages of sound field systems. The major companies that sell sound field technologies are listed in Appendix A at the end of this chapter.

CLASSROOM OBSERVATION

The first consideration in attempting to improve acoustical conditions in a classroom is to determine what is desirable and what is feasible within a particular room. Refer to Chapter 9 for more information about classroom observation. Also important is that audiologists survey the acoustic conditions of the classroom and make determinations as to how best to solve unacceptable acoustic conditions. Methods for acoustical modification of the classroom are discussed in detail in Chapter 7.

Certainly, the first step in sound field placement is the systematic reduction of classroom noise and reverberation. Unfortunately, even after extensive room modifications, many classroom environments will still not meet recommended criteria. Consequently, because of the excellent cost-benefit ratio of sound field amplification, use of this method alone may be the only feasible solution in a particular situation. Clearly, the additional S/N ratio enhancement provided by sound field amplification can compensate for the loss of speech energy over distance and benefit every student in the classroom. In short, as discussed in Chapter 1, the installation objective for sound field amplification systems is to improve the S/N ratio about 10 decibels for each student location in the classroom.

WIRELESS MICROPHONE MODALITY

Until recently, virtually all sound field classroom amplification systems used wireless microphones based on frequency modulation (FM) radio technology.

TABLE 8-1   Advantages of sound field amplification

- The system can be used with each of the populations of normal-hearing children as well as children with SNHL. As indicated in this book, the vast majority of children in our school systems can benefit from sound field amplification.
- In terms of children with mild SNHL, the system can provide some benefit while malfunctioning hearing aids or auditory trainers are repaired.
- Sound field systems are often the most inexpensive procedure for improving classroom acoustics. Certainly, as discussed in Chapter 1 and here in Chapter 8, such systems are the least expensive of the assistive listening devices used for classroom amplification.
- A sound field system does not stigmatize certain children, which can be the situation with auditory trainers or hearing aids because they require the children to wear hardware.
- Most teachers willingly accept sound field amplification systems. Moreover, teachers report lessened stress and reduced vocal strain during teaching activities.
- Students can utilize the system's pass-around microphone for oral reports, oral reading, and for asking and answering questions, thus enhancing academic performance and their own auditory-feedback loop.
- Sound field systems can be used to enhance other instructional equipment (e.g., televisions, cassette tape players, CD players).

TABLE 8-2   Potential disadvantages of sound field amplification

- Sound field amplification systems may not provide adequate benefits in excessively noisy or reverberant learning environments. That is, 8–10 dB of amplification may not be enough to overcome the effects of a particularly poor acoustical environment. Specifically, the use of sound field amplification can increase both the level of the desired direct sound and the undesired reflected sound energy. In addition, because of varying amounts of sound cancellation and distortion, obtaining the desired uniform sound amplification throughout the classroom may be difficult.
- If the loudspeaker arrangement is not appropriate for the classroom, the teacher's voice may be amplified excessively for some children while not providing sufficient amplification for other children. In both situations, the benefits to the student and teacher will be diminished.
- In smaller classrooms, the amplified sound may be less than 10 dB because of feedback problems associated with the synergistic effects of reflective surfaces and speaker closeness. At present, how much benefit limited amplification can provide is not clear.
- Both the teacher and the student need appropriate in-service information and follow-up support for the sound field system to provide maximum benefit in the classroom.
- Sound field amplification cannot be used as a substitute for personal FM systems for children with more than very mild degrees of hearing loss.

This technology is reliable and has historically served to enhance the S/N ratio in thousands of classrooms. With a sound field FM system, the microphone converts an acoustic voice signal into an electrical signal that, in turn, frequency-modulates a carrier frequency. The frequency-modulated carrier frequency is what the wireless microphone broadcasts. A receiver demodulates (separates) the original speech signal from the carrier signal; the original signal is then amplified and delivered to loudspeakers. Unfortunately, FM technology has several limitations that have frequently prevented full implementation of sound field amplification in many classrooms and school systems. The limitations primarily relate to the limited number of separate carrier frequencies on which to transmit a signal, spillover of signal transmissions close in frequency, and interference of the transmitted wireless microphone radio signals.

FM Interference

Since the advent of the use of FM wireless microphones in amplification systems, the number of separate frequencies has been an issue. Because FM wireless microphone radio transmissions can travel significant distances and because these signals can penetrate solid structures such as walls and ceilings, FM-based systems set to the same frequency can potentially transmit and receive other signals. It is obviously not acceptable for students in one classroom to hear a different teacher transmitting from another classroom on a different subject. In order to solve this problem, wireless microphones and receivers are set to separate carrier frequencies so that a classroom transmission can only be received in that classroom. Unfortunately, there are a limited number of clear carrier frequencies available for classroom use, so the number of separate classrooms that can use wireless microphones in a school is constrained. In some applications, where the number of classrooms to be amplified does not exceed the available clear frequencies, this constraint will not be a factor. In an effort to increase the number of separate frequencies, manufacturers have set transmitters close to each other in frequency. This solution is not perfect, because when frequencies are close together there is the potential for loss of fidelity and interference, much like when you tune a radio just off the active frequency. Other frequencies close by also can be picked up, thus distorting the wanted signal.

Unfortunately, FM frequencies are not exclusive to classroom use, so there is a potential in some locations to pick up nearby powerful FM broadcasts from radio stations or police and emergency services, especially when the teacher's transmitting microphone is turned off. In addition, the FM signal itself can be distorted in transmission based on orientation of the antenna and electromagnetic sources in the classroom or building. Since the purpose of installing sound field FM technology is to improve the S/N ratio in the classroom, thereby facilitating attention and acoustic accessibility of instructional information, intermittent static, buzzing, clicking, random conversations, or unwanted music transmitted over the sound field loudspeakers is obviously not desirable. In recent years, some manufacturers have started using higher carrier frequencies in an effort to increase the number of available clear channels. In the final analysis, the successful use of an FM sound field system depends on factors such as number of classrooms to be amplified and availability of clear carrier frequencies in the school area.

Infrared Transmission

In order to overcome the primary FM wireless microphone limitations, infrared (IR) wireless microphones have been introduced into many sound field amplification systems. In these systems, an acoustic signal is used to frequency-modulate a carrier frequency that, in turn, amplitude-modulates infrared light-emitting diodes. The amplitude-modulated infrared light is broadcast to the receiver that houses infrared photodetectors and necessary demodulators. The original acoustic signal is recovered, amplified, and delivered to loudspeakers in the room.

Since light cannot penetrate solid surfaces such as walls and windows, the transmitted signal is largely confined to the room in which the wireless microphone is used. Because the signal is confined to a particular classroom, there is no need for alternative frequencies to separate signals from adjacent classrooms. Therefore, there are no constraints on the number of classrooms that can be amplified within a building, and all of the wireless microphones are likely to be compatible across the entire school system. In addition, outside interference from disruptions by electromagnetic sources and other FM signal broadcasts is virtually eliminated.

Infrared systems, however, are not without possible problems. Interference from sunlight, fluorescent lights, and other light sources can make some IR systems difficult or impossible to use. In addition, the infrared light emitted by the transmitting microphone must be able to be received by the photodetectors in the receiver. To achieve this, care must be taken to set up the IR system so that the light path is unobstructed and materials in the room do not absorb the infrared light spectrum. Lack of attention to these issues will lead to signal dropout and interruptions of the amplified sound through the system. Table 8-3 provides a brief comparison of FM and IR sound field technologies.

COST FACTORS

Sound field systems vary in price from about $800 to more than $2,000 depending on the type of system (infrared can be a little more expensive).

TABLE 8-3   Comparison of FM and IR sound field systems

Concern	FM	IR
Number of frequencies	Limited	Unlimited
Interference/Distortion	Possible from other transmissions on same frequency	Possible from sunlight or other infrared sources
Signal dropout	Usually not an issue	Can be a problem
Multiple microphones	Possible but each microphone must be on a separate frequency, which further reduces available frequencies	Provision for two micro phones—no effect on nearby systems

Quality of equipment, number of loudspeakers, service contracts, ease of installation, durability, flexibility, and such special features as an extra transmitting microphone for team teaching all impact the cost. Like it or not, school systems are operating on tighter and more restricted budgets. See Chapter 11 for ideas about how to market and obtain funding for sound field systems.

Cost is mentioned here not only to acknowledge its importance, but also to introduce a caution. Evaluating *all* of the issues relative to selecting and installing sound field systems, and not just the cost of the equipment, is important. We certainly want the best-quality sound system for the lowest price. However, be aware that a low-fidelity system that is not user-friendly, has significant interference, or often breaks down with no warranty or service contract can be far worse than not having any sound field equipment at all. A thirty-day trial period represents a reasonable amount of time to evaluate cost-effectiveness.

CARRIER FREQUENCIES

Different equipment manufacturers may use different frequency bands in their wireless microphone system. Frequency is more of an issue in FM systems, so we shall first address radio frequencies.

We do not recommend constructing a sound field system from off-the-shelf audio components. There are many pitfalls in the use of these constructed systems. A short list of possible pitfalls includes use of frequencies susceptible to inference, very limited carrier frequency selection, no provision for additional microphones, too much battery drain to last a full school day, inadequate loudspeakers, poor quality, and lack of customer service and support.

Sound field FM equipment typically uses VHF (very high frequency) or UHF (ultrahigh frequency) carrier frequencies. Frequency bands that are used for low-power FM transmission for individuals with hearing impairment include 72–76 MHz and 216–217 MHz. These frequencies tend to have the least interference, lower transmission range, and lower cost. Recently, higher UHFs such as 900 MHz have been employed in sound field systems. Whatever band is used can be subdivided in order to increase the number of discrete channels within the band (which determines how many systems can be used simultaneously). The 72–76 MHz band, for instance, can be broken down into ten wide-band channels of 200 Hz each or forty narrow-band channels of 50 Hz each. The narrower the band, the greater the chance for distortion due to diminished fidelity, reduced S/N ratio, and reduced modulation headroom (Boothroyd, 1992).

In the past, IR carrier frequencies were standard. This meant that most any IR system would work with any other IR system in production. Recently, however, other IR carrier frequencies have been introduced, so compatibility of systems is now an issue. This is a particularly important consideration if you are adding a newer IR system in a school that has an older IR system in place. Of course, if the IR system will only be used in a specific classroom, compatibility may not be a concern. Because of the introduction of new FM and IR carrier frequencies, some companies have developed translators that can transpose and match carrier frequencies between systems and thus compatibility. The Microfield and Auto Pilot devices manufactured by Phonak are examples of recently developed translators; others are in the experimental phase at this writing.

NUMBER AND POSITIONING OF LOUDSPEAKERS

How many loudspeakers and where to place them are probably the most frequently asked questions when considering a sound field amplification system. Unfortunately, these are the questions that can be answered with the least certainty. We need more data-based studies to investigate these issues because of the many geometric and acoustic variables present in each individual classroom environment. Classroom variables include size, shape, construction materials, and seating arrangements. Learning styles also vary considerably: whole-group versus individual learning, versus small-group interactive learning, versus learning centers, versus independent learning, versus self-contained classrooms, versus open classrooms. Teaching style is another important variable and includes single-teacher lecture, team teaching, or multiple teaching occurring simultaneously at several learning centers through-out the room. The students themselves add yet additional variables according to their ages, numbers in a class, compliance, and any disabling conditions they may possess. Refer to Chapter 9 for more information about this issue.

Would the same sound field loudspeaker arrangement be suitable for the plethora of classroom compositions, teaching styles, and pupils just men-tioned? Probably not! To the contrary, amplifying an auditorium or a theater is relatively easy to achieve by following a fixed formula, because the stage is always up front, the actors and speakers are always on the stage, and the spec-tators are always seated in stationary chairs in fixed positions throughout the room.

In the past we have recommended taking a pragmatic approach to order-ing and installing sound field equipment. This pragmatic approach consid-ers the individual classroom, the individual teacher and teaching style(s) used in it, and the pupils who learn in that particular classroom. Recently, a simu-lation approach has been advocated that holds great promise of resolving many of the unknowns in speaker placement.

The Simulation Approach

Simulations are used in architectural acoustics to estimate the impact of acoustic modifications before the modifications are actually made. Using this approach, a series of *what if* scenarios can be computed and the best modifi-cations selected for a particular room. Siebein, Crandell, and Gold (1997) have shown that by measuring the impulse response of a room, the acoustic characteristics of the room can be documented and used in calculations to predict speech perception.

Recently, a classroom acoustics simulation has been developed for use in choosing and placing sound field components in a classroom (Boothroyd, 2000). The Phonic Ear Sound Field Wizard is a shareware program that can be downloaded from the Phonic Ear Web site (www.phonicear.com). This useful program allows the user to input certain physical characteristics of a classroom (room dimensions, background noise level, reverberation time), the location of the teacher in the room, location and characteristics of sound field loudspeakers within the specified room, and important variables (ear height of listeners, distance of microphone, and gain of the sound field sys-tem). From this information, calculations are made and reported graphically on a grid of the specified classroom. Most student seating locations can be found on the grid. At each grid-location signal level, S/N ratio, audibility index, phoneme errors, word-in-isolation errors, and word-in-sentence errors can be calculated and displayed. The mean and ranges for each calculated parameter are also displayed so that comparisons between grid locations can be made. By experimenting with the program's input parameters, you can obtain the best estimated student performance for each location on the grid. Determinations can easily be made concerning the impact of loudspeaker characteristics, such as height and location within the room, but as you can see, many other decisions concerning speech perception can also be made.

While not all room configurations and not all commercially available loudspeakers are represented in the program, the simulation is a very useful tool. One caveat in using simulation programs is that any simulation will be based on assumptions and philosophies of the programmers. Be sure that you agree with the assumptions and philosophies. Remember, too, that simulations produce estimates; actual measurements may vary from the estimates. Currently, we recommend experimenting with simulation programs and using them in conjunction with the pragmatic approach. With additional data-based studies, simulation programs are likely to take on greater importance and use in selection and placement of sound field systems.

The Pragmatic Approach

Loudspeaker Placement Objectives

Remember, the primary acoustic issues in a classroom are signal-to-noise ratio and reverberation. To improve S/N ratio, we can increase the intensity of the signal, reduce the intensity of the noise, or both. As stated earlier, an emerging role for the audiologist is to be an advocate for reducing background noise levels through acoustic modifications. Sound field amplification is used to increase the intensity of the signal.

A typical design goal for a sound field system is to increase the signal intensity about 10 dB uniformly throughout the classroom. In order to accomplish this, we must know something about the room and something about the loudspeakers used in the sound field system. First, one must realize that reverberation can either help or hinder speech perception. Late room reflections (about 50 msec caused by reflections from distant surfaces in the classroom) interfere with the speech signal and are considered noise. However, earlier reflections add to the original speech signal and actually increase the intensity of the original signal. By placing the student close to a loudspeaker, two goals are accomplished: the intensity of the signal is increased by amplification, and addition of noise by late reverberation is avoided because the student only receives early reflections. Desktop or toteable sound field systems have been introduced to provide these ideal sound field conditions for individual students. Figure 8-1 depicts a small loudspeaker placed on a student's desk. Usually, students with exceptional listening needs, such as those with cochlear implants or at high risk for listening problems, use this new form of sound field amplification. Obviously, not all students in the room benefit from

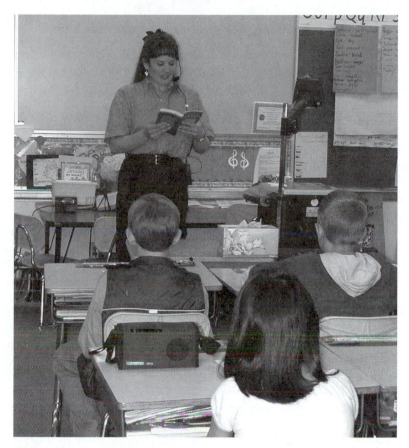

Figure 8-1. A small loudspeaker (personal sound field system) placed on a pupil's desk can increase the loudness of the teacher's speech and enhance early reflections. (Photograph courtesy of LightSPEED Technologies.)

this kind of system because it does not provide uniform amplification throughout the classroom.

Determining the Number of Loudspeakers

Adequate acoustic dispersion of the teacher's voice throughout the classroom is a function of many factors, including the wattage of the sound field amplifier used, the directionality of loudspeakers, and the location and number of loudspeakers in the room. Using multiple loudspeakers has been common practice in order to accomplish adequate dispersion, although there is little research to base this decision on anything other than intuition and what sounds good to the installer. As is well recognized, carelessly installed multiple loudspeakers in a room can alter the acoustic spectrum of the talker's signal and may produce psychoacoustic effects such as listener fatigue. Single point speakers may have fewer problems, but they may not allow for an even distribution of sound throughout the room.

There is some evidence that four or more loudspeakers installed and distributed in the ceiling provide the best dispersion of sound to all in the room. Some different loudspeaker designs, such as bending wave flat panel and high directivity, may provide more options. Because new speaker designs hold the promise of higher fidelity and less loss of speech energy, they may well be the speaker designs of choice in the future (Prendergast, 2001). More research is needed in this area to ascertain the best way to accomplish adequate dispersion of speech energy in classrooms.

Obviously, the goal is for all students in the learning field to have access to an even, consistent, and favorable S/N ratio at a 10 dB improvement over unamplified speech. Thus, if group learning is the mode of teaching, the entire classroom needs to be amplified evenly; all the pupils need to be able to hear the teacher at all times. The larger the classroom, typically the greater number of loudspeakers (three or four) that need to be used so that each child is closer to a loudspeaker than he or she could be to the teacher. Close proximity avoids loss of critical speech elements as the sound signal is transmitted across a physical space. If angled properly, three or four loudspeakers positioned about five feet up on walls or in a ceiling array could provide surround sound for all students.

If the classroom has learning centers, a loudspeaker could be positioned close to each learning center for maximum effective amplification of the critical locations. If only one learning center is used at a time, then the other loudspeakers should be turned off.

If a small resource classroom is used, two loudspeakers could provide an even and consistent S/N ratio throughout the area. In fact, if the room is quite small, and there are only a few students who can be seated close to the teacher, even a single loudspeaker might be effective.

If the classroom and class size are small with only one teacher-instructed learning center in use at any given time, then the teacher could carry a single battery-powered loudspeaker to each teaching location to amplify that specific environment. This single portable loudspeaker arrangement has worked very effectively in some preschool settings.

Figure 8-2 shows the use of a single portable loudspeaker to amplify a learning center. This particular teacher does not use a group instruction paradigm. Rather, all instruction is carried out in small learning centers, and the teacher carries the battery-powered loudspeaker with her to each individual location. This particular loudspeaker uses infrared rather than FM transmission.

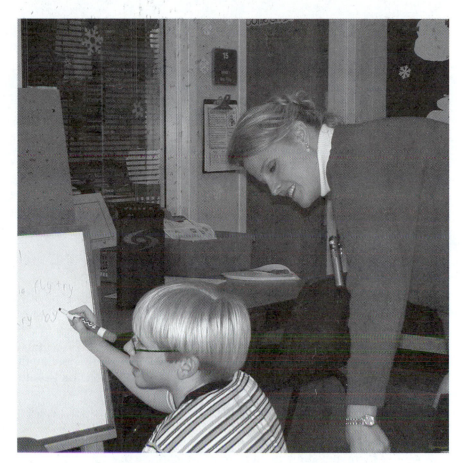

Figure 8-2. A single, portable, battery-powered infrared loudspeaker can be easily moved by the teacher to amplify a particular learning environment. (Photograph courtesy of LightSPEED Technologies.)

Loudspeaker Positioning

Unfortunately, there are no data-based guidelines for loudspeaker placement. Again, a pragmatic approach is recommended. It seems logical that sound could be heard most efficiently if it is directed to the ears of the children. Consequently, some manufacturers recommend placement of loudspeakers on speaker stands at the ear level of children. The problem with such placement is that the stands tend to get knocked over by active young children or obstructions occur between the loudspeaker and the ears of children. Other manufacturers recommend placing loudspeakers at several feet above the ears of seated children with the loudspeakers angled downward. For many reasons, the authors have found greater success with this latter recommendation.

The speaker angle of dispersion is certainly an issue. Some teachers, in a practical effort, place loudspeakers on any available bookshelf, facing any which way. Other teachers mount the loudspeakers up high on the walls toward the ceiling. Loudspeakers that are mounted high on walls can cause increased room reverberation if the sound is bounced off the ceiling.

Loudspeakers inadvertently have been turned backwards or have had gerbil tanks, books, or other obstructions placed in front of them. Loudspeakers must remain unobstructed and angled toward the children. The point is that loudspeakers that are not thoughtfully placed can cause more reverberation in a room rather than overcome a poor acoustic environment. Loudspeakers placed in ceilings also need to be unobstructed and angled to allow a favorable angle of dispersion.

Loudspeaker Output Measurement

Refer to Chapter 6 for suggested measurement protocols and worksheets. Measurement strategies include making sound-level measurements; obtaining rapid speech transmission index (RASTI) scores; and subjectively evaluating the sound of the unit, called ear cuing. Speech that is heard through a sound field system should be easily and uniformly audible from and at all learning locations in the classroom. In addition, spoken instruction should be comfortably intelligible and not stressful.

An empty classroom might sound very different from an occupied classroom. That is, we typically install a sound field unit in an empty room. When students arrive with their sound absorbent bodies and their noise-generating abilities, the sound field unit might need to be readjusted.

DURABILITY, FLEXIBILITY, PORTABILITY, AND EASE OF INSTALLATION OF SOUND FIELD EQUIPMENT

Some sound field loudspeakers are intended to be permanently installed on the walls or in the ceiling of a particular room, while others need to be moved to other rooms or within a room as seating arrangements and learning centers change. Questions that need to be asked include: How user-friendly is the equipment? How heavy are the loudspeakers? How flexible is the speaker wire? How many hands do you need to transport the equipment? How robust is the sound field equipment? Equipment that is fickle or fragile is of no value to anyone. Does the equipment break easily? How quickly can repairs be made? Are loaner parts available? Is there a trial period? How supportive is the manufacturer?

OVERALL FIDELITY OF THE SOUND FIELD SYSTEM

Issues to consider include the quality of the microphone, amplifier electro-acoustic characteristics, and the loudspeaker frequency response and dispersion characteristics. We also need to be mindful that room acoustics shape the acoustic signal and interact with the sound field system. The specification sheets for the sound field system components can be quite different in different rooms. It appears that a high-frequency emphasis signal enhances the intelligibility of speech and enables children to detect word-sound differences (Flexer, Millin, & Brown, 1990). More research is needed to determine how much of a high-frequency emphasis is needed.

Listen to the equipment. Does it crackle? Does the signal sound like it is on the verge of feedback when set to a comfortable listening level? Are there "hot spots" where feedback occurs if the teacher walks near certain areas in the room?

A sound field system is meant to be a valuable teaching tool that facilitates classroom instruction, thereby enhancing learning. If equipment malfunctions in any way, sounds "weird," or interferes with teaching, teachers likely will turn off the unit rather than fix the problem.

PLACEMENT OF A CHILD WITH A KNOWN HEARING IMPAIRMENT

Technically, sound field enhancement amplifies the entire classroom to a relatively constant level. However, we know that sound is degraded as it is propagated away from the source (Leavitt & Flexer, 1991). Therefore, continuing with our pragmatic orientation, it seems logical to seat the child who has a known hearing problem (typically minimal, mild, unilateral, or fluctuating) close to one of the loudspeakers (for sound enhancement) and close to the teacher/media materials (for visual enhancement). Since we are on the subject of children with hearing loss in the classroom, one question often asked is whether it is feasible to use a sound field unit and personal FM system together in the same room. This issue is addressed in the next section.

Using Sound Field Systems and Personal FM Systems in the Same Classroom

Questions arise about using personal FM systems and sound field systems together in the same classroom. Is one better than the other? Should personal-worn FM and sound distribution systems be used at the same time? Can personal-worn FM and sound distribution systems be used at the same time? Does the teacher need to wear two microphones? At this point, it is critical to emphasize that sound field systems are not replacements for personal-worn

FM systems. Most children who wear hearing aids or cochlear implants continue to need the superior S/N ratio provided by personal-worn FM systems that channel the signal directly from the talker through the hearing aids or cochlear implant to the brain of the listener.

However, both sound field distribution systems and personal FM systems can be used effectively in the same room. In many instances, using both at the same time can create the best listening and learning environment because each serves a different purpose. The sound field system, appropriately installed and used in a mainstream classroom, improves and equalizes acoustic access for all pupils and creates a quieter listening environment in the room. Moreover, if the teacher has been appropriately in-serviced, she employs the vocal strategies of using a softer and more interesting voice (Rosenberg et al., 1999). In addition, she will implement listening strategies that benefit everyone in the room. Another substantial advantage is that static or system malfunction is noticed by all. When there is only a personal FM system in use in a classroom, only the child who is wearing the FM receiver hears static; thus, system malfunction can last for days or weeks (Ross, Brackett, & Maxon, 1991).

The individual-worn FM system allows the particular child with a hearing aid or cochlear implant to have the most favorable S/N ratio. The teacher need wear only a single microphone or transmitter if the sound field unit and the individual FM are on the same radio frequency—or if the personal-worn FM transmitter can be coupled to the sound field amplifier as shown in Figure 8-3.

A significant advantage to integrating a personal-worn FM system with a classroom sound system, as shown in Figure 8-3, is pupil access to the pass-around microphone of the sound field system. Most sound field systems use two microphones—one for the teacher and the second to be passed around to whomever is speaking, as shown in Figure 8-4.

A personal-worn FM system has access to only one microphone—the teacher's. If the personal FM transmitter is coupled to the sound distribution system, as shown in Figure 8-3, the child will hear pupils speaking through the pass-around microphone as well. The two microphones will provide the child who wears a hearing aid or cochlear implant plus a personal-worn FM system with much greater access to classroom information.

WHAT TYPE OF MICROPHONE SHOULD THE TEACHER WEAR?

Microphones used in sound field systems are meant to be placed within six inches of the sound source. If they are placed farther away, off axis, or on noisy movable surfaces such as necklaces, sound distortion results. Typical microphone styles include lavaliere, collar, or boom (head-worn) types. The boom or head-worn microphone seems to offer the most consistent signal because

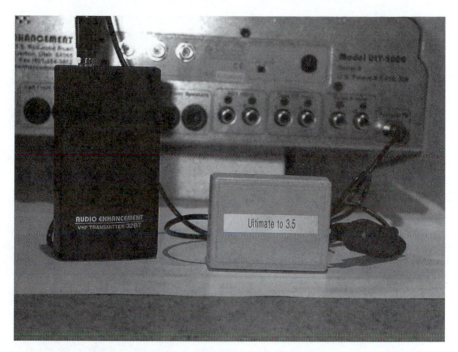

Figure 8-3. The transmitter of a personal-worn FM system can be coupled, via an appropriate cord, to a specified jack, or audio-output port, of a sound field system. With this arrangement, the teacher need wear only the transmitter of the sound distribution system, and the child who wears the personal FM system will have access to both the teacher's transmitter and the second pass-around microphone that accompanies the sound field system. (Photograph courtesy of Audio Enhancement.)

the microphone turns when the teacher's head turns. The disadvantage of this setup reported by teachers is that it can be uncomfortable.

NECESSITY OF A POINT PERSON

A critical variable for the effective installation and use of sound field equipment is the presence of a support or contact person within or easily available to the school district who can install the equipment, present in-service training, and monitor equipment function and use. Classroom amplification systems represent a significant change for school systems, both in operation and philosophy; that change requires a facilitator. Without a facilitator or support person, sound field equipment might not be used or might not be used efficiently.

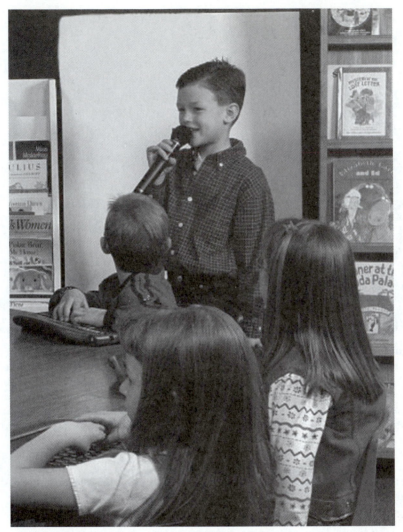

Figure 8-4. The pass-around microphone of the sound field distribution system allows all pupils to have enhanced access to classroom information. (Photograph courtesy of Audio Enhancement.)

ACOUSTIC FEEDBACK CONTROL

Acoustic feedback in a sound field system occurs when the amplified signal from a loudspeaker is picked up via the wireless microphone and is then reamplified. This reamplification of sound creates system oscillation, which perceptively results in a "howl" or "squeal" to the listener. Acoustic feedback with sound field amplification can occur when (1) the teacher is positioned too close to a loudspeaker; (2) the gain, or volume of the system, is set too high; (3) or both. Thus, to avoid feedback, loudspeakers must be positioned so that the teacher can be within any instructional area in the classroom but not in close proximity to the loudspeaker. Loudspeakers positioned in the ceiling, elevated on the walls, or in noninstructional areas can fulfill this objective. In addition, highly directional loudspeakers can assist in acoustic feedback reduction.

To reduce the potential of acoustic feedback in the classroom, it is also imperative that the gain of the sound field system not be set beyond levels that would amplify the teacher's voice by more than 8–10 dB. Gain settings that provide levels in excess of this can result not only in feedback, but also in reductions in signal quality. The gain of a sound field system also can be increased (i.e., the potential of acoustic feedback can be reduced) by decreasing the distance from the teacher's mouth to the microphone (a boom microphone is particularly useful in reducing this distance) or by using a highly directional microphone. A unidirectionally wired microphone could also be used to reduce acoustic feedback; however, such a setup will restrict teacher mobility (Berg, 1993).

Operationally, the maximum gain of a sound field unit (before reductions in quality or feedback occur) can be determined via the following formula (Berg, 1993):

$$\text{Maximum Gain (in dB)} = 20 \text{ Log } D_o - 20 \text{ Log } D_s + 20 \text{ Log } D_1 - 20 \text{ Log } D_2 - 6 \text{ dB}, \tag{8.1}$$

where D_o = distance from the speaker to the listener, D_s = distance from speaker to the microphone, D_1 = distance from the loudspeaker to the microphone, and D_2 = distance from the loudspeaker to the listener. Thus, if we assume that D_o (distance from the speaker to the listener) is 20 feet, D_s (distance from speaker to the microphone) is 0.5 feet, D_1 (distance from the loudspeaker to the microphone) is 5 feet, and D_2 (distance from the loudspeaker to the listener) is 10 feet, we develop the following equation for maximum gain:

$$20 \text{ dB Maximum Gain} = 20 \text{ Log } 20 - 20 \text{ Log } 0.5 + 20 \text{ Log } 5 - 20 \text{ Log } 10 - 6 \text{ dB} \tag{8.2}$$

Technologies developed in the proaudio field are finding their way into sound field systems. Some of these technologies include digital signal processing (DSP) algorithms to reduce acoustic feedback, thereby allowing greater amplification of the acoustic signal.

ROLE OF THE AUDIOLOGIST

In the past, sound field amplification was considered a remedy for acoustic conditions that affected students at risk for listening and learning problems.

Because these children were often designated as requiring special education services, the audiologist in the school was often closely involved with decisions concerning sound field amplification. However, due to research showing that sound field amplification can benefit all students in a classroom as well as the teacher, sound field amplification is more and more considered a regular education element that may or may not include the audiologist in the decision-making cycle for installation of sound field amplification. The role of the audiologist thus changes from a fitter of the technology to the person responsible for establishing efficacy of the technology. This is a familiar role for audiologists and is necessary to ascertaining the effectiveness of installations of sound field equipment, whether installed as part of a special education or regular education program.

SUMMARY

This chapter has presented many issues to consider when amplifying a classroom. A pragmatic approach is recommended, but the reader should be on the lookout for new simulations that may be useful. The goal of sound field amplification is to provide an even and consistent S/N ratio improvement of approximately 10 dB throughout the learning area. The learning area to be amplified depends on the physical layout of the classroom, the listening demands placed on the pupils, and the teacher's individual instructional style. The reader is referred to Appendix B for use and maintenance tips for sound field amplification systems and to Appendix C for troubleshooting tips.

DISCUSSION TOPICS

1. Discuss the objectives of placing sound field amplification in a classroom.
2. List the advantages and disadvantages of FM and infrared sound field amplification systems.
3. List the most common troubleshooting issues when using a sound field amplification system.
4. Discuss what is meant by pragmatic and simulation approaches to installation of sound field amplification systems.
5. How can sound field amplification be used with other technologies designed for children who are deaf or hard of hearing?

REFERENCES

Berg, F. (1993). *Acoustics and sound systems in schools*. Clifton Park, NY: Thomson Delmar Learning.

Boothroyd, A. (1992). The FM wireless link: An invisible microphone cable. In M. Ross (Ed.), *FM auditory training systems: Characteristics, selection and use.* Timonium, MD: York Press.

Boothroyd, A. (2000). *The sound field wizard.* Phonic Ear Web site, www.phonicear.com.

Flexer, C., Millin, J. P., & Brown, L. (1990). Children with developmental disabilities: The effect of sound field amplification on word identification. *Language, Speech and Hearing Services in Schools, 21,* 177–182.

Leavitt, R., & Flexer, C. (1991). Speech degradation as measured by the rapid speech transmission index (RASTI). *Ear and Hearing, 12,* 115–118.

Prendergast, S. (2001). A comparison of the performance of classroom amplification with traditional and bending wave speakers. *Journal of Educational Audiology, 9,* 1–7.

Rosenberg, G. G., Blake-Rahter, P., Heavner, J., Allen, L., Redmond, B. M., Phillips, J., & Stigers, K. (1999). Improving classroom acoustics (ICA): A three-year FM sound field classroom amplification study. *Journal of Educational Audiology, 7,* 8–28.

Ross, M., Brackett, D., & Maxon, A. (1991). *Assessment and management of mainstreamed hearing-impaired children.* Austin, TX: Pro-Ed.

Siebein, G., Crandell, C., & Gold, M. (1997). Principles of classroom acoustics: Reverberation. *Educational Audiology Monograph, 5,* 32–43.

APPENDIX 8-A
SOUND FIELD AMPLIFICATION MANUFACTURERS

Anchor Audio, Inc.
3415 Lomita Blvd.
Torrence, CA 90505
800-262-4671
www.anchoraudio.com

Audio Enhancement
14241 South Redwood Road
Box 2000
Bluffdale, UT 84065
800-383-9362
www.audioenhancement.com

Comtek Communications Technology, Inc.
357 West 2700
Salt Lake City, UT 84115
800-496-3463
www.comtek.com

Custom AllHear Systems, Inc.
20325 28th Avenue West
Lynnwood, WA 98036
800-355-7525
www.customallhear.com

Lifeline Amplification Systems
41 Means Drive, Suite A
Platteville, WI 53818
800-236-4327
www.lifelineamp.com

LightSPEED Technologies, Inc.
11509 SW Herman Road
Tualatin, OR 97062
800-732-8999
www.lightspeed-tek.com

Phonic Ear, Inc.
3880 Cypress Drive
Petaluma, CA 94954-7600
800-227-0735
www.phonicear.com

Sennheiser Electronics Corporation
1 Enterprise Drive
Old Lyme, CT 06371
877-736-6434
www.sennheiserusa.com

TeachLogic
22984 Triton Way, Suite C
Laguna Hills, CA 92653
800-588-0018
www.teachlogic.com

Telex Communications, Inc.
Educational Products
12000 Portland Avenue South
Burnsville, MN 55337
800-328-3102
www.telex.com

APPENDIX 8-B
USE AND MAINTENANCE TIPS
FOR SOUND FIELD TECHNOLOGIES

- Handle the equipment carefully to avoid bumping, jarring, or dropping.
- Avoid placing the equipment in areas of excessive cold or heat, such as in direct sunlight.
- Avoid placing equipment in areas where it might be damaged by water, excessive dust, or moisture (e.g., near an open window, sink, or aquarium or near the chalkboard).
- Each morning, remember to turn on the receiver or amplifier and transmitter/microphone and check the operation of the system. If there is no sound, decreased volume, or poor sound quality, use the troubleshooting checklist to identify the problem.
- Do not cut, pin, or staple through the microphone connector cord or the speaker wires.
- Remember to turn off all equipment (transmitter/microphone and receiver or amplifier) at the end of each day.
- Remember to charge the transmitter each night. (Do not charge disposable batteries, as they may rupture and damage the unit.)
- Remember to insert batteries with the correct polarity (+ to + and – to –).
- Position the transmitter face down on a cushion or other soft surface when removing and inserting batteries.
- Provide a dust cover to protect the microphone or transmitter and receiver or amplifier at night and over weekends and holidays.
- Periodically clean the equipment with a soft cloth. Do not spray any cleaning agents on the equipment.

APPENDIX 8-C
TROUBLESHOOTING SOUND FIELD SYSTEMS

No FM reception (NO FM light stays on)
1. Verify that the frequency code number of the transmitter/microphone and the receiver or amplifier are the same.
2. Verify that the frequency selector switch is set correctly.
3. Check battery's charge and polarity (+ to + and – to –). Recharge or replace the transmitter batteries.
4. Verify that the antenna is properly connected to the antenna jack on the receiver or amplifier.
5. Contact the audiologist if you have checked all of the above and the NO FM light remains illuminated.

No sound
1. Check items 1–4 under "NO FM reception."
2. Verify that the receiver or amplifier is turned to the on position.
3. Verify that the transmitter is turned on.
4. Check connections between receiver or amplifier and wall transformer.
5. Plug the receiver or amplifier into a different wall outlet.
6. Verify that loudspeaker wires are connected to the receiver or amplifier and loudspeaker terminals.
7. Verify that loudspeaker wire leads are not touching each other at the loudspeaker or the receiver or amplifier terminals.
8. Check the microphone connector cord for damage. (Wiggle the cord to determine if wires have been damaged.)
9. Contact the audiologist if you have checked all of the above and there is still no sound from the system.

Weak loudspeaker output
1. Recheck wiring to make sure cables are connected in phase.
2. Recharge or replace battery.
3. Check the receiver or amplifier volume control setting(s).
4. Reposition microphone closer to the talker's mouth.
5. Realign loudspeakers if they have been moved so that they are no longer directed toward the students.
6. Contact the audiologist if you have checked all of the above and the system continues to have weak loudspeaker output.

Poor sound quality
1. Replace battery.
2. Check battery prong connections in the transmitter and charger unit. (The + and – connections in the battery compartment and the charger unit need to be periodically tightened to ensure proper contact.)

3. Verify that the antenna is properly attached to the receiver or amplifier.
4. Check the loudspeaker wires for cuts or poor connections.
5. Check the microphone connector cord for damage. (Wiggle the cord to determine if wires have been damaged.)
6. Check the volume control settings on the receiver or amplifier.
7. Contact the audiologist if you have checked all of the above and the system continues to exhibit poor sound quality.

Feedback
1. Lower the FM volume control setting on the receiver or amplifier.
2. Increase the distance between the loudspeaker(s) and the transmitter microphone.
3. Contact the audiologist if you have checked the above items and the system continues to feed back.

FM interference
1. Contact the audiologist and describe the type of interference noted (e.g., paging system, security system, other classroom conversation, etc.)
2. A different FM frequency will need to be selected for the classroom in the event of interference from another broadcast source. An infrared system may be necessary to eliminate radio interference.
3. The receiver or amplifier will need to be reset to accommodate the change in transmitter frequency.

CHAPTER 9

From System Selection to Enhancement of Listening Skills: Considerations for the Classroom

Carolyn Edwards, MClSc, MBA

KEY POINTS

- There are various types of classroom settings including closed, open concept, split grade, and portable that all may require a different type of sound field system as well as different placement and use.
- Sound field systems are most effective in classrooms where didactic teaching and a single talker are the norm.
- The type of activities conducted in a classroom and the amount of time spent on each will determine if a sound field system can be effectively used as well as determine the need for single-channel or dual-channel capability; the number of loudspeakers and type of loudspeaker arrangement suited to the learning style of the classroom; the type of microphone required; the hardware modifications or accessories necessary, if any; and recommendations for implementation of the system during daily activities.
- Installation of the sound field system should be done with special consideration of the safety of the students and the best possible location for amplification to be effective.
- Sound field systems can be beneficial in many ways; for example, they can assist teachers who experience vocal fatigue.
- If the speech signal is optimized using sound field FM or infrared technology plus additional teaching strategies in the classroom, chil-

dren can direct their finite amount of energy to processing and comprehending the speech signal, thus capitalizing on what the teacher is there to offer educationally.

- It is important for the audiologist to follow up with teachers and students after installation to ensure that they are properly using the system and benefiting from the amplification.
- Many students and teachers aren't aware of the distractions, noise, and bad acoustics of a room that are interfering with their learning until the sound field system in the room has been removed after being used for an extended period of time.
- Both teachers and students should share responsibility for monitoring noise-level control in the classroom.
- When sound field FM or infrared technology is introduced simultaneously with a focus on the development of listening skills and strategies, acoustic enhancement of the signal will be optimized.

Sound field systems become a part of the learning environment from the moment they are introduced into the classroom. It is vital to recognize the potential impact of classroom amplification systems on the teacher, the class, and the classroom structure and routines in order to ensure appropriate installation, maintenance, and use of the systems by teacher and students. This chapter will review factors for consideration in the introduction of a sound field system into a classroom, from candidacy and selection to enhancing listening skill development.

TYPE OF CLASSROOM

There are many types of classrooms including closed, open concept, split grade, and portable.

Closed Classroom

There are a variety of classroom styles used in the educational setting. The most traditional format is the closed classroom, where each classroom is a separate room in the school building. This situation allows for the simplest installation for sound field systems and use of the system as it was originally designed.

Open Concept

Open concept areas became popular in the 1980s and continue to be used in a number of school districts. The purpose of open concept classrooms is to permit team teaching, cross groupings of children between classes, and movement of children among classrooms without physical barriers. Up to eight classes could be located in the same physical space without any walls to separate the classes. Enhancement of the speech signal is highly desirable since the speech-to-noise ratios are often poorer than closed classrooms, for two reasons: the background noise levels are predictably higher, and the teachers often use softer than average voice levels in order to reduce interference with the teachers in adjacent classes. However, use of sound field systems in these environments is quite challenging and may be impossible in some sites. Teachers in open concept areas using sound field systems need to coordinate schedules with teachers in adjacent classes so that they are not using the sound field system at the same time. Otherwise, the enhanced signal from one class simultaneously interrupts students listening to their teacher in the adjacent area. Where wall or table loudspeakers are used, face the loudspeakers into the individual teaching area, away from the other classes. Classes at opposite ends of the open teaching areas may be able to utilize amplification without any problems. Given the necessity to modify schedules and work together, teachers' acceptance and willingness to experiment are essential for successful introduction of sound field systems in these settings.

Split Grades

When there are insufficient numbers of students to form a class of a single grade, schools may combine two grades in one classroom with a single teacher. Teachers in split grade classrooms tend to teach one grade while the other grade is working on small group or independent activities, and generally each grade is physically grouped together in the classroom. In this situation, one does not want to amplify the teacher's voice during a lesson to both grades at the same time. It is therefore desirable to use sound field systems where loudspeakers can be turned off in the part of the room the teacher is not using or alternately where the teacher can carry the loudspeaker(s) to the area where she or he will be teaching in the room.

Portable Classroom

In schools where the enrollment has far exceeded the original capacity of the school, portable classrooms have been installed. Portables are stand-alone installations outside the school building with separate ventilation and heating systems. Unfortunately, the hollow floors, which are designed to enhance portability, produce greater reverberation than a solid floor, and often the rooms are uncarpeted, leading to increased noise levels from the sound of chairs and desks scraping on the floor. I measured an intensity level of 84 dB (A) from the sound of one chair scraping on the floor of a portable. Naturally, teachers tend to use louder voices to compensate for the poorer acoustic conditions, resulting in more rapid vocal fatigue than that experienced by teachers within the school building. Therefore, the benefits of sound field systems for teachers in portable classrooms are readily apparent. Teachers in portable classrooms report an immediate decrease in their vocal intensity with the introduction of a sound field system and a resulting decrease in vocal fatigue.

CLASSROOM SEATING

The type of classroom seating adopted by the teacher is a matter of teaching style and students' ages. In the younger grades where interactive learning approaches are favored, teachers may create up to six activity centers in the room where small groups of children rotate in and out, and children circle around the teacher for large group activities. The ideal amplification for activity center formats is a portable loudspeaker that the teacher can carry. An option for multiple speaker systems is an off/on toggle switch installed in the wiring or on the loudspeaker of some units; the teacher can turn the loudspeaker on when talking to children in that particular activity center and turn the loudspeaker off when leaving the activity center so that children in other activity centers do not receive the amplification. Large group instruction with young children often occurs within only one part of the classroom; positioning of single or multiple loudspeaker systems must ensure that loudspeakers provide a satisfactory teacher signal during large group instruction, in addition to amplifying activity centers. In the older grades where didactic approaches are more common, row seating is typical and there are fewer variables to consider in loudspeaker placement.

TEACHING STYLE

The need for a sound field system is dictated by the learning styles favored by the classroom teacher. Teachers may use one or more of the following approaches: didactic large or small group activities, interactive large or small group teacher-directed activities, interactive small group activities monitored by the teacher, and individual work.

Didactic Teaching Style

Individual FM systems were originally designed in the early 1970s when didactic approaches were the standard in education. Thus, the concept of a single transmitter worn by the teacher sending a one-way speech signal to the student was appropriate. However, despite changes in teaching practices, which began to incorporate activity-based experiential learning, traditional FM system design has not changed radically. Sound field systems are most effective in classrooms where didactic teaching and a single talker are the norm.

Interactive Teaching Style

To maximize the benefit of sound field systems in interactive large or small group teacher-directed activities, the use of a pass-around microphone (see Chapter 8, Figure 8-4) or a second transmitter on a separate frequency to amplify students' voices in discussion is ideal and is an excellent way to teach talker and listener strategies. The teacher must be prepared for a slower pace of discussion to accommodate physically passing the microphone to the student speaking. This is only viable, however, in primary or junior grades where the children are grouped around the teacher in close proximity. It is usually not feasible to pass the teacher transmitter from child to child in the row-seating arrangement seen in the older grades. Use the pass-around microphone or the second transmitter on a separate frequency. Where the pass-around microphone option is not available, passing the teacher transmitter from child to child during discussion is desirable. Note that the teacher's voice will not be amplified while the transmitter is being passed among the students. The other alternative is to have the teacher repeat a student's answers through the teacher transmitter so that the answers are amplified for the whole class.

Small Group

There are several considerations in use of the sound field system during small group activities monitored by the teacher. Teachers can carry their transmitters from group to group; however, amplifying the children's voices for each other once the teacher leaves the group is problematic when using sound field systems. This is unfortunate since peer discussion is often a primary avenue for learning in many classrooms.

If the sound field system has been placed in the classroom specifically for a child with hearing loss, the teacher may wish to leave his or her transmitter with the small group in which the particular child has been placed while ensuring that other loudspeakers in a multiple loudspeaker system are turned off. Of course, the teacher is then unable to present an amplified signal to any of the other small groups.

Teachers can use the transmitter and carry a portable loudspeaker to that location or turn on the speaker (using the switch on the speaker wire or on the speaker) in the vicinity of the small group when they are talking to the group in order to amplify their voices. Discuss with teachers how they interact within small group activities; often the amount of commentary by the teacher visiting each of the small groups is limited. It is possible that the educational audiologist and the teacher may decide not to amplify speech during these small group activities. If so, then the number of suitable loudspeaker options expands considerably.

Team Teaching

Two teachers will sometimes combine classes together in one room and teach together. Given that two transmitters cannot transmit on the same frequency without creating interference and also given the limitations of passing one transmitter back and forth between two teachers, the manufacturers have created several options to address this scenario.

- Single-channel sound field system with hand-held microphone on same channel (Teacher 1 must turn her transmitter off each time Teacher 2 speaks); second teacher transmitter on same channel (same conditions as above).
- Single-channel sound field system and personal FM system (with two-channel transmission) daisy chain arrangement whereby a sound field system is coupled with a personal FM system in the following way: Teacher 1 wears transmitter 1 (personal FM system) and transmits to Teacher 2 who wears receiver 1 (personal FM system) patched in through the audio out-jack on the receiver to the audio in-jack on transmitter 2 (sound field system), which then transmits to the amplifier and subsequently to the loudspeakers in the class.
- Dual-channel sound field FM or infrared system transmitter where transmitters 1 and 2 are used on different channels at the same time without interference.

Independent Work Periods

As children move into higher grades, teachers may assign projects requiring independent efforts to research, design, and write. It is important to determine how much time is spent in these kinds of activities; in one classroom I visited, 90% of classroom time was dedicated to individual student projects. Use of a sound field system in this classroom may not be warranted.

CANDIDACY AND SELECTION OF SOUND FIELD FM SYSTEM

It is helpful to sit down with the teacher and draw up a schedule of the type of activities conducted in the classroom and the length of time spent in each type of activity. (See Appendix 9-B for recording form.) This information will determine if a sound field system can be effectively used; whether single-channel or dual-channel capability is needed; the number of loudspeakers and type of arrangement suited to the learning style of the classroom; the type of microphone required; the hardware modifications or accessories necessary, if any; and recommendations for implementation of the system during daily activities.

PREPARING CLASSROOM TEACHER FOR INSTALLATION AND USE

The use of classroom space reflects the individual teaching style of each teacher. Some spread the students' desks throughout the room, others group the desks together and use the remaining space for activity centers and storage, and others set aside some space for children to work, read, or reflect on their own. It is more difficult to install loudspeakers in a classroom partway through the school year when the teacher has already designed the layout of the room. Meeting with the classroom teacher at the outset of the year allows the audiologist to become familiar with the classroom traffic flow and gives the teacher the opportunity to make changes in floor plans that increase the ease of speaker installation. Many manufacturers recommend locating amplifiers not integrated into the loudspeakers away from any computers in the classroom to reduce interference issues. Table-mounted loudspeakers and speaker stands should be secured to ensure physical safety of the students. Ceiling loudspeakers should be located in the center of the teaching space, not necessarily the center of the classroom. Certain loudspeakers should be located approximately three feet from the corners of the room to reduce reflection. Where a single loudspeaker is used in the classroom, the choice of location of the speaker should be carefully considered based on the nature of the activities within the classroom. Loudspeakers should not be located in "dead space" where no instruction occurs or close to areas set aside for quiet time where children go to avoid the bustle of the classroom. Wiring for loudspeaker systems can be routed through a dropped ceiling or around the tops of chalkboards and doors to eliminate any wiring close to the floor. Amplifiers should be located away from the classroom sink and preferably away from the main traffic flow of the students. Often the location of electrical outlets limits choices considerably. There must be space provided above the amplifier to permit extension of the antenna.

Creation of a Receptive Attitude

Successful introduction of sound field systems is dependent on teacher receptivity to the concept of amplification and to follow-up provided by support personnel. Teachers are often encouraged by the reports of improved listening and an increased rate of instruction attributed to less need for repetition seen with students in classes using sound field systems. However, typically it is not talking about sound field systems that persuades classroom teachers to experiment. Generally, demonstration and actual usage are the factors that provide convincing evidence.

Although changes in students' behaviors take some time to observe, the most obvious change in the first few minutes of use is the reduction in the teacher's vocal intensity. Depending on the subject area taught, the background noise levels in the class, and individual personalities, some teachers are at higher risk for vocal fatigue than others. Teachers in the primary grades who provide only oral instruction all day long, such as in foreign language classes, have often reported laryngitis a few weeks after school begins. Physical education teachers can easily abuse their voices when attempting to project in highly reverberant and noisy gymnasiums. Access to a demonstration system is the most effective way to show teachers the benefits of enhancing signal for student listening and reduction of teacher vocal fatigue.

Issues in Acceptance of the System

Teachers' primary resistance, if any, to sound field amplification is the use of the hardware and the reluctance to be "on the air" throughout the day. Use of a boom microphone, which improves the signal significantly on many sound field systems, may initially be undesirable for comfort or cosmetic reasons for some teachers. When sound field systems were first introduced, there was only one design for a boom microphone and many teachers found it uncomfortable. Now there are a variety of designs for boom and collar microphones on the market that provide for variation in head size and shape as well as use of eyeglasses. When the sound field system is being installed, it is useful to bring several different models for teachers to try on so that they can select the boom microphone most comfortable for them. Consideration of comfort issues during the installation creates a better environment for acceptance of the system. Also useful is demonstrating the difference in sound quality among boom, collar, and lapel microphones so that the teacher recognizes the benefits of the boom microphone.

The ease of use of the transmitter overcomes the resistance of most teachers to the hardware. The audiologist's job is to make the loudspeaker choices and placements simple and practical for the teacher to implement. Unlike personal FM systems, remembering to turn the transmitter off during conferences with individual children is an easy matter with sound field systems since the teacher immediately hears the amplified signal within the room. However, there have been cases reported of teachers forgetting to turn their transmitters off when going to the staff room. Students gathered around the loudspeakers in the classroom with great glee to listen to the private discussions of staff members.

Once installed, there are some teachers who may not use the system as much as desired during the day; they comment that the children don't "really need" the amplification during particular activities. Further in-service training may provide more reinforcement to increase consistency of use.

Key Points during In-Service Training

In-service training with all teaching staff prior to using the sound field system is important to overcome the attitude that students can hear adequately in the classroom without amplification. Refer to Chapter 1 for information about content of in-services.

Because students have lived for many years with a poor signal in a poor acoustic environment, many teachers assume that students cope satisfactorily. Yet, the fatigue that children develop in a poor listening environment has received little attention to date from audiological researchers. It is reasonable to assume that children in poor acoustic environments must expend considerable energy simply extracting the speech signal. If the speech signal is optimized using sound field FM or infrared technology and additional teaching strategies in the classroom, children can direct their finite amount of energy to processing and comprehending the speech signal, thus capitalizing on what the teacher is there to offer educationally. Therefore, the message that must be conveyed to teachers during in-service training is that although many children appear to cope with difficult listening environments, amplification of the teacher's speech enhances children's learning potential.

The most effective in-service tool used by the author to demonstrate the effect of reduced hearing on perception of speech is the simulation of hearing loss using foam earplugs. (See suggested outline for a hearing loss simulation in Appendix 9-C.) This experience gives teachers personal insight into the strains of listening under poor acoustic conditions. The increased ease of listening offered by sound field systems is also strongly supported in anecdotal reports. It is therefore encouraging to new users to include during in-service training other teachers who already use the system and can discuss their experiences. When all has been said and done, I have not found one teacher or class that has wished to discontinue using a sound field system once it has been installed and comprehensive in-service training and follow-up services have taken place. The following is a list of effective in-service tools:

- Simulation of hearing loss
- Demonstration of the sound field system
- Reports from other teachers who are experienced users of sound field systems
- Reports on the impact of noise on understanding of speech in children
- Research reports showing the impact of sound field systems on educational performance of children in the classroom

Follow-up after Installation

Installation of the system is only the first step in enhancing listening skills in children. Follow-up is essential to sustain the focus on listening skills in the classroom. Visiting the classroom on a monitoring basis maintains the visibility of hearing in general and the sound field system specifically. Visitation also permits ongoing discussion of any issues arising about usage. Once the teacher is comfortable with using the transmitter, the audiologist should encourage the children to participate in the use of the system. Once the audiologist demonstrates good microphone technique to the students, they can practice passing the transmitter among themselves during discussions. This not only enhances perception of the children's voices but also teaches children good talker-listener strategies, which the teacher can carry over to all other classroom activities.

Selection, installation, in-service, and follow-up of sound field systems is a detailed process involving the collaboration of the educational audiologist, the teacher, and the children in the classroom. When the variables affecting the learning environment are understood, systems can be selected and used appropriately, and the benefits for children's learning are substantive.

ENHANCEMENT OF LISTENING SKILLS IN THE CLASSROOM

With every new amplification option, there is the technical element and the human element. The introduction of sound field systems into the classroom provides a new technology to enhance the listening environment. The introduction of new and thoughtful teaching strategies to improve the listening environment and students' listening abilities can maximize the use and benefit of technology.

Listening is the primary avenue for teaching and peer learning in the classroom. Optimal listening skills develop in an atmosphere that supports the enjoyment of sound, communication, storytelling, and experimentation. An ideal listening environment includes activities such as the following:

- sharing ideas and feelings
- listening centers where children can listen to music and taped stories
- daily storytelling by teacher and children
- children creating their own theater and plays
- singing or playing simple musical instruments
- experiments with sound, such as creating new sound effects for a ghost story
- science experiments with sound, such as the effects of different sounds on plant growth

The term "listening" in its broadest context means responding to, organizing, interpreting, and evaluating sound in order to create meaning (Early Childhood Curriculum Committee, 1978). In other words, listening is the ability to detect, discriminate, identify, and comprehend various auditory signals. Detection is the ability to respond to sound, pay attention to sound, and learn not to respond when there is no sound. Discrimination is the ability to attend to differences among sounds, or to respond differently to different sounds. Identification is the ability to name or identify the sound heard. Comprehension is the ability to answer questions, follow instructions, paraphrase, or participate in a conversation (Erber, 1977).

The sense of hearing is used for several purposes: to comprehend the speech of others, to monitor our own speech, and to monitor the surrounding environment (Edwards, 1991). The focus of listening activities in early childhood curricula, however, is often comprehension of speech only. There is little or no discussion of strategies to enhance the environment in which students listen, despite the evidence that noise and reverberation have a deleterious effect on children's comprehension (Crandell & Smaldino, 1996; Finitzo-Hieber & Tillman, 1978; Johnson, 2000; Neuman & Hochberg, 1983; Picard & Bradley, 2001; Yacullo & Hawkins, 1987).

There are many different aspects of listening in the classroom. Activities recommended in this section will focus on the following:

- increase student and teacher awareness of the listening environment
- change the listening environment
- enhance talker-listener skills when faced with more difficult listening conditions

Making Sound Visible

Development of listening skills starts first with awareness of sounds that exist within the classroom environment. The first step is to make sound and specifically noise "visible" in the classroom. Although classroom noise is obviously interfering, teachers and students often adapt and accept noise as a normal characteristic of the classroom environment. In a study completed in schools in Quebec, Canada, 54% of classroom teachers and 77% of physical education teachers reported that noise usually caused communication problems in their respective work environments, in contrast to only 9% of office workers interviewed (Hétu, Truchon-Gagnon, & Bilodeau, 1990). Despite such data, there are no consistent efforts to reduce noise levels in the classroom. While there are acoustical standards to stipulate maximum allowable noise levels to prevent noise-induced hearing loss in school building codes and recommended acoustical standards for the design of new classrooms, there is no legal mandate regarding noise levels in school buildings. There continues to be limited recognition of the impact of noise on children's learning within educational circles.

Placement of a sound field system in the classroom is often the first opportunity teachers and students have to experience an improvement in speech-to-noise ratio. The change in the environment created by the new technology can provide the impetus for enhancing awareness of noise in the classroom.

Once the sound field system has been in place for about two to three weeks, have the teacher turn the system off for part or all of one day. Then, have the children record their observations and consider the following questions:

- Are there any noises they notice that they hadn't noticed before? Are there any differences in the sound? If so, what are they?
- Is the noise level in the classroom softer or louder than before?
- Are they having difficulty hearing the teacher?
- Can they remember if they had difficulty hearing the teacher before the system was installed?

Have the teacher answer the following questions:

- Does the teacher use a louder voice when the system is off?
- How do the children respond to instructions?
- Does the teacher have to repeat more?
- Is there a longer transition time between activities when the system is off?
- What is the background noise level in the classroom now?

The contrast between amplification and no amplification is an excellent experience to heighten students' awareness of typical speech and noise levels in the classroom. Graduate students in speech-language pathology and audiology were completing a one-week course in educational audiology that I taught in a room they had used as a lecture hall for the past two years. A sound field FM system was installed for the week to provide them with firsthand experience of room amplification. At the end of the week when the system was turned off during discussion period, the students complained about the poor room acoustics, a factor that previously had never attracted their attention.

Using a sound-level meter is another way to increase awareness of noise. Several electronics distributors sell an inexpensive sound-level meter that schools can purchase. Students in third grade or higher can easily learn to use a sound-level meter to measure sound occurring in the classroom. Prior to measurement, it is instructive to have students estimate the loudness of the sound in decibels with a simple rating scale such as quiet, average, a little loud, and very loud, so that they begin to develop a comparative sense of sound intensities. Later teachers can ask the students to rate the noise levels based on the degree of interference with communication and work, using a simple scale such as quiet, slightly interfering, moderately interfering, extremely interfering, and too loud to communicate or work independently. Students are often surprised to discover the loud intensity level of sounds such as fans from the ventilation system or the recess bell.

Encourage students to measure any sounds of interest occurring in the classroom, and notice if students become more aware of room noises as a result of the ongoing measurement of sounds. Teachers can also ask the students to measure sound levels in other parts of the school and report to other classes or teachers about the results. These reports can create an opportunity to in-service others. Audiotaping the classroom at different times of the day can provide the students with more information about speech and noise levels in the class.

Teachers can experiment with a "silent" half-day or full day where no sound is permitted. The only allowable communication is through gesture, drawing, or writing, and students are asked to keep all classroom sounds to a minimum. Paradoxically, it is often only when noise is reduced or eliminated that students and teachers become aware of its presence in the room. Usually after the experience of a silent day, students are more aware of noises that exist in their classroom and, more specifically, the noises they themselves generate.

Teachers and students in the classroom frequently ignore the sound of chairs scraping on uncarpeted floors. Ask each student to bring in two pairs of socks, and attach the socks with elastic bands to the bottom of the each student's chair legs to reduce the noise generated by chair movement. After two weeks, remove the socks and have the students report their observations. Did they notice a difference? How loud is the sound of the chairs moving? Can they hear what other students are saying when someone moves a chair at the same time? Again, note that the auditory experience is heightened by experimenting first with the absence of the noise and then returning to the original condition. (You can substantially decrease noise from chairs scraping on the floor by placing precut tennis balls on the bottom of the chair legs for the duration of the year. See Appendix 9-C for a newsletter article for teachers about the use of tennis balls for noise reduction.)

It is also important for students to be aware of the differences in teachers' and classmates' speech levels as a function of distance and intensity levels. Some students may have difficulty hearing the classroom discussion adequately when they are sitting at a distance from the talker or when listening to students who do not project their voices well. Passing the transmitter of the sound field system during class discussion often permits some students to be heard and understood for the first time. If students are unaware of differences in intensity in their voices, measure the loudness of other students' voices through the loudspeakers using the sound-level meter. One can never overdo awareness exercises. To maintain the "visibility of sound," it is useful to repeat activities such as the ones described here throughout the school year.

Changing the Environment

When teachers and students have a greater awareness of noise or poor quality speech signals, they are ready to initiate changes in the listening environment.

After using the sound field system for a few weeks, encourage daily monitoring of appropriate use by the students. For example, have the teacher start the day without the system turned on and wait for the students to notice. The teacher may do this from time to time and reward the student who first notices that the system is turned off. When the students pass the transmitter around during class discussion, ensure that the child does not begin to talk before receiving the transmitter. In classrooms using row seating, students in the seats at the back of the classroom are often the first to notice a poor signal during large group discussions where the microphone cannot easily be passed among the children. Encouraging students to say "I can't hear you" sets up a more proactive attitude toward listening expectations when students are sharing ideas.

When the sound field system is not in use, the teacher can assign a student to act as voice monitor for the day. The monitor's responsibility is to ask the speaker of the moment to talk louder, more clearly, or both. Although the sound field system enhances the speech signal, monitoring and decreasing noise levels is a function best suited to the teachers and students in the classroom. The difficulty to date in any technological means of removing noise is that noise is defined by the person listening, not by a set of acoustical parameters (Boothroyd, 1994). For example, what is considered noise from several students working together to the student reading to himself at an adjacent table is the primary speech signal for the students in that group. Noise is any speech or environmental sound that interferes with the individual's ability to focus on the task at hand.

Monitoring noise levels usually has been the prerogative of the classroom teacher. However, since students create the majority of the noise within a classroom, it is appropriate for students to share along with the teacher responsibility for noise control (Melancon, Truchon-Gagnon, & Hodgson 1990). In my experience, assigning students responsibility for noise control has worked very effectively in a number of classrooms. The power of the student monitor to ask classmates to be quiet is very motivating for most students. Through the earlier work measuring sound levels with the sound-level meters, the students should be able to maintain some consistency in their estimation of excessively loud sound. At a more sophisticated level, students in some of the higher grades have formed committees to evaluate noise in the classroom and report back to the class with a set of recommendations for noise control. A hearing conservation program could also add some complementary information, particularly for young teenagers at risk for noise-induced hearing loss. The National Institute on Deafness and Other Communication Disorders (NIDCD) Information Clearinghouse offers a free unit for school children on hearing conservation.

Setting aside an area of the classroom for quiet times also reinforces the teacher's support for noise reduction. Teachers have often used old bathtubs or a mound of pillows to create a "castle" or cocoonlike area where the students can go to read or work on their own without talking. In one classroom, the quiet area called "The Office" was in such demand that there was a line to get in! Giving students opportunities to make changes in their listening environments can create advocates for better acoustics.

Talker-Listener Skills

Use of the sound field system is an excellent way to teach talker and listener skills. Good microphone technique is the first talker skill that teachers and students can practice with sound field systems. The teacher can experiment with various locations of the boom or lapel microphone, with respect to clarity and intensity of her or his speech. Involving the students in determination of optimal placement of the microphone gives them an opportunity to develop finer auditory discrimination and recognition skills. Subsequently, the students can experiment with the appropriate microphone distance for optimal sound quality.

With or without amplification, talkers and listeners can disrupt or distort the message. Students need practice in identifying behaviors that are characteristics of good talkers such as facing the listener, speaking clearly, and indicating the beginning and ending of a remark. Characteristics of good listeners include facing the speaker, acknowledging the speaker's comments, and waiting until the speaker is finished talking. Students also need to observe the characteristics of poor talkers and listeners. By using role-playing where the talker's voice is amplified through the sound field system, the whole class can participate in evaluating, from appropriate to poor, speaker and listener behaviors. Of course, students' favorite parts are always the bad talkers or listeners.

Modeling unclear messages teaches the children different ways that they interfere with communication. Using the sound field system as a simulation of communication on the telephone, the transmitter can be passed back and forth between two students. The teacher gives one student secret instructions about how to make his or her message more difficult to understand, and the rest of the students have to guess how the student is distorting the message.

The sound field system can be used in any number of comprehension activities to enhance the talker's voice. Use of the teacher transmitter during storytelling, children's theater creations, and singing provides better amplification of the children's voices to each other, resulting in more optimal communication.

Development of Listening Skills in the Classroom

Sound is an invisible characteristic of classroom conditions. Activities that encourage teachers and students to respond to, organize, interpret, and evaluate sound increase visibility of sound. Sustained visibility is the most important factor. Rather than complete many of the suggested activities during the first few weeks that the sound field system is introduced, it is better to introduce one activity per week and extend the focus on listening strategies throughout the year. For example, during the first week, the teacher may work on microphone technique with the students. In the second week, the students may be asked to measure specific noises that occur in the classroom. The following week, the teacher may ask the students to bring in some socks or tennis balls for the chair legs. Later, the students may do a science experiment measuring various noises outside the school. The continued focus on listening activities and sound is a constant reminder of the importance of hearing and, specifically, the importance of high-quality speech input.

Follow-up is an essential part of any activity in order for the skill to become part of classroom routines and children's listening practices. Have the children create posters in the room to remind them of various lessons, such as the characteristics of good talkers and listeners. For the younger children, puppets can remind them of the behaviors of good speakers and listeners. When someone in the class is not listening well, the classroom teacher can ask the other students to suggest ways in which the poor listener could improve in that moment. Students serving as noise monitors build in awareness of noise levels in the class on an ongoing basis. Encouraging students to acknowledge and search for possible reasons for listening difficulties during daily activities focuses attention on ways to change the listening environment.

MAXIMIZING THE USE OF THE SOUND FIELD SYSTEM IN THE CLASSROOM

Encourage students to use the sound field system during any sharing time, announcements, or presentations to the class. This is generally not difficult since children of any age like to talk into a microphone. Teachers can amplify any of the audio or audiovisual sound sources such as record players, tape recorders, film projectors, and videocassette recorders, either by placing the microphone beside the sound source or patching directly into the transmitter, which is possible on some systems. All teachers working with the class, including the foreign language, music, or art teacher, should receive a complete in-service so that they, too, can use the sound field system effectively.

SUMMARY

When sound field FM or infrared technology is introduced simultaneously with a focus on the development of listening skills and strategies, acoustic enhancement of the signal will be optimized. A one-shot approach to listening programming will not make a difference. Only the systematic inclusion of listening into everyday activities and ongoing explorations into various aspects of listening will enhance the auditory development of children in the classroom.

DISCUSSION TOPICS

1. What are important points to remember when preparing a classroom teacher for installation and use of a sound field system?
2. What are different types of microphones that can be used or worn by the teacher?
3. List and describe three effective in-service tools.
4. What are the purposes of the sense of hearing?
5. Briefly discuss one awareness activity that can be useful for maintaining the "visibility" of sound.
6. What are characteristics of a good listener?

REFERENCES

Boothroyd, A. (1994). Hearing aids. Paper presented at Technology for Communication and Education Symposium, Rochester, NY.

Crandell, C., & Smaldino, J. (1996). Speech perception in noise by children for whom English is a second language. *American Journal of Audiology, 5*(3), 47–51.

Early Childhood Curriculum Committee. (1978). *Listening and speaking.* Adelaide: Publications Branch, Education Department of South Australia.

Edwards, C. (1991). Assessment and management of listening skills in school aged children. *Seminars in Hearing, 12*(4), 389–401.

Erber, N. (1977). Evaluating speech perception ability in hearing impaired children. In F. Bess (Ed.), *Childhood deafness: Causation, assessment, and management.* New York: Grune and Stratton.

Finitzo-Hieber, T., & Tillman, T. (1978). Room acoustics effects on monosyllabic word discrimination ability of normal and hearing impaired children. *Journal of Speech and Hearing Research, 21*, 440–458.

Hétu, R., Truchon-Gagnon, C., & Bilodeau, S. (1990). Problems of noise in school settings: A review of the literature and the results of an exploratory study. *Journal of Speech-Language Pathology & Audiology, 14*(3), 31–39.

Johnson, C. (2000). Children's phoneme identification in reverberation and noise. *Journal of Speech, Language and Hearing Research, 43*(1), 144–157.

Melancon, L., Truchon-Gagnon, C., & Hodgson, M. (1990). *Architectural strategies to avoid noise problems in child care centres.* Montreal, Canada: Groupe d'acoustique de l'Universite de Montreal.

Neuman, A., & Hochberg, I. (1983). Children's perception of speech in reverberation. *Journal of the Acoustical Society of America, 73*, 2145–2149.

Picard, M., & Bradley, J. (2001). Revisiting speech interference in classrooms. *Audiology, 40*, 231–244.

Yacullo, W., & Hawkins, D. (1987). Speech recognition in noise and reverberation by school-age children. *Audiology, 26*, 235–246.

APPENDIX 9-A
RESOURCES FOR DEVELOPING LISTENING SKILLS

The following are additional recommended resources for developing listening skills:

125 Ways to Be a Better Listener
By N. S. Graser (1992)
Published by Linguisystems, Inc., East Moline, Illinois

Sound Science
By E. Kaner (1991)
Published by Kids Can Press, Ltd., Toronto, Ontario

Listening: A Basic Connection
By M. Micallef (1984)
Published by Good Apple, Inc., Carthage, Illinois

APPENDIX 9-B
SAMPLE FORM TO DETERMINE CLASSROOM REQUIREMENTS

Type of Activity	Length of Time	Teacher Involvement	Use of Sound Field and Loudspeaker Placement
Morning Schedule			
Afternoon Schedule			

Recommendations:

Use of sound field system	Yes _____ No _____
Type of speaker arrangement	Portable _____ Fixed _____
If fixed, type of speakers	Ceiling _____
	Wall mounted _____
	Table mounted _____
Number of speakers:	1 _____
	2 _____
	3 _____
	4 _____
Type of microphone	Boom microphone _____
	Collar microphone _____
	Pass-around microphone (same frequency) _____
	Pass-around microphone (different frequency) _____
Modifications required	Yes _____ No _____
Describe modifications	
Accessories required	

- Patch cord for personal FM transmitter
- Patch cord for audiovisual equipment
- Extra batteries
- Extra boom microphone for use with students
- Belt for transmitter

APPENDIX 9-C
SIMULATION OF HEARING LOSS:
AN INSERVICE TRAINING TOOL

Direct experience often produces optimum learning. Most teachers who are faced with the prospect of a child with hearing loss in their classroom for the first time, express concern about their ability to address the child's needs in their class. By giving the teacher some direct experience with hearing loss, you can provide them with

- an empathetic understanding of the communication demands on the child with hearing loss in the classroom.
- an understanding of the teaching strategies that are detrimental to communication in the classroom.
- an understanding of the teaching strategies that are beneficial to the child with hearing loss in the classroom.

Use of foam earplugs can simulate a mild conductive hearing loss of approximately 25 to 35 dB. The following points are important to emphasize to school staff.

- The simulation only creates a mild hearing loss, and so students with moderate, severe, or profound hearing loss will experience greater difficulty than that experienced with the earplugs.
- The simulation reflects what children with mild hearing loss may hear without a hearing aid, or what children with moderate or moderately severe hearing loss may hear with the hearing aid on.
- Use of the earplugs simulates a conductive rather than a sensorineural hearing loss, since the earplugs are simply impeding the passage of sound through the external ear. This is an important distinction, since the staff must realize that the distortion of speech sounds and the susceptibility to noise seen with children with sensorineural hearing loss cannot be simulated through the use of earplugs alone.
- The simulation produces an accurate perception of the hearing loss often seen with children with recurrent otitis media. Although many teachers may not have experiences with children with sensorineural hearing loss, all primary teachers will have a number of children in their classes each year with histories of recurrent otitis media. (Otitis media is the single most common reason for a child to visit the family physician, and the most common cause of hearing loss in children.)

Suggested Procedure

After explaining the purpose of the exercise, hand out a pair of foam earplugs to each group member. Ask the participants to hold the plugs by the rounded edge and roll them between their fingers to compress them to approximately 1/3 to 1/4 of their original size.

Then have everyone insert the compressed plugs into their ear canals so that the canals are completely occluded. If the participants do not hear a clear difference in the loudness of the sound after inserting the plugs, the plugs have not been inserted correctly. Have the individuals remove and reinsert the earplugs. Then ask the participants to get out a sheet of paper and pencil to write down what you say. *There are a number of concepts that you want to demonstrate during the simulation.*

- The farther away the speaker is from the listener, the more difficult the listening task.
- Restricting speechreading cues makes the listening task more difficult.
- Presence of background noise increases the difficulty of the listening task.
- The type of material presented will vary the difficulty of the task. Single words are much more difficult to identify than is sentence material, where contextual clues can provide a great deal of information.
- The intensity of vowels is greater than that of consonants, thus increasing the ease of vowel recognition.
- High frequency consononants such as /s/, /f/, /ch /, /k/, /t/, and the voiceless /th/ are usually the most difficult sounds to hear, particularly the /f/ and voiceless /th/, since they are the softest of all of the consonants.
- Listening under difficult conditions is fatiguing, resulting in a tendency to tune out or daydream.
- Listening can be very frustrating when speakers are far away, or are covering their mouth, or when background noise is present. The listener may experience anger or frustration towards the speaker or towards the sources of background noise.
- Additional visual supplements such as writing on the blackboard or the overhead projector can be of great assistance in following the conversation, and reduce the strain of listening.

Ask participants to write numbers 1 to 15 on the side of the page. In order to demonstrate the above concepts, present words and sentences in the following way.

Write the word....

    1. please   BY HEARING ALONE
    2. great   (MOUTH COVERED);
    3. sled   QUIET CONVERSATIONAL LEVEL;
    4. pants   MOVE AROUND WHILE YOU ARE
    5. rat   TALKING

Write the word.....

    6. bad   BY HEARING ALONE
    7. pinch   (MOUTH COVERED);
    8. such   CREATE BACKGROUND NOISE
    9. bus   (PAPERS RUSTLING, KEYS JINGLING,
  10. need   BOOK DROPPING ON FLOOR.....);
                 QUIET CONVERSATIONAL LEVEL;
                 MOVE AROUND WHILE YOU ARE
                 TALKING

Write the word....

  11. ways   BY HEARING AND SPEECHREADING
  12. five   (MOUTH UNCOVERED);
  13. mouth   QUIET CONVERSATIONAL LEVEL;
  14. rag   BACKGROUND NOISE SPORADIC
  15. put

Now ask the participants to number their page from 1 to 10 and tell them that you will now say some sentences.

    1. Walking is my favorite exercise.
    2. Here's a nice quiet place to rest.
    3. Somebody cleans the floors every night.
    4. It would be much easier if everyone would help.
    5. Open your window before you go to bed.
            BY HEARING ALONE
            (MOUTH COVERED);
            BACKGROUND NOISE SPORADIC
    6. Do you think that she should stay out so late?
    7. How do you feel about beginning work at a different time every day?
    8. Move out of the way.
    9. The water is too cold for swimming.

10. Why should I get up so early in the morning?
       BY HEARING AND SPEECHREADING
       (MOUTH UNCOVERED);
       BACKGROUND NOISE SPORADIC

- It is important to use a quiet conversational voice level rather than a normal conversational level for maximum effect.
- Because sentences are considerably easier to identify than are single words, they are presented through hearing alone in noise, rather than in quiet.
- The background noise can be sporadic or continuous; the listeners will experience the frustration in either situation.
- When moving around, ensure that you rotate around the entire room so that everyone can experience both optimal and least desirable listening conditions.

Then have the participants take up their answers WITH THE EARPLUGS STILL INSERTED. When a person gives his or her answer, ensure that the rest of the group has heard it. If not, ask the person to change the way that he or she has presented the answer so that others will understand better (such as repeating the response, saying the word or sentence louder, facing the group, spelling the word, or adding an accompanying gesture). Write down the various answers on a chartboard or overhead to provide a visual supplement. Underline the correct answer from all of the choices provided by the participants.

Once all of the words and sentences have been reviewed, HAVE THE GROUP TAKE OUT THE EARPLUGS. Initiate a group discussion of the following issues:

- their emotional reactions to the overall experience.
- the causes of specific frustrations experienced.
- insights about the experiences of children with hearing loss in the classroom.
- ways in which they could change their teaching strategies to address the needs of children with hearing loss.

The discussion deepens the experience of the simulation of hearing loss and allows participants themselves to determine the necessary changes in teaching strategies.

APPENDIX 9-D
TENNIS BALLS INCREASE CHILDREN'S ATTENTION

Carolyn Edwards, MClSC, MBA

Children hear more poorly than adults in noisy situations. Although there is a gradual improvement through the elementary years, children are thirteen to fifteen years of age before they can cope in noise as well as adults do. Children with recurrent ear infections, language disorders, English as a second language, hearing loss in one ear, or any degree of hearing loss in both ears have even more difficulty than their peers understanding speech in noise.

Classrooms are noisy places, and the noise is primarily generated by children talking and chairs moving on uncarpeted floors. To give you an idea of sound levels, teachers' voices are often at a loudness level of 65 dB SPL. During activity times, loudness levels range from 70 to 85 dB SPL. The sound of one chair scraping on the floor of a portable classroom was measured at 85 dB SPL. (The sound of a motorcycle or a jackhammer is about 100 dB SPL.)

Noise interferes with children's comprehension of speech. Studies have consistently shown decreases of 35–40% in children's speech recognition from a fairly quiet room to the typical noise levels experienced in today's classroom.

Tennis balls are an inexpensive way to decrease chair noise in the classroom. To make your own sound absorbers, take an Exacto knife and cut an X in the top of each tennis ball. The X should be just large enough to insert the metal leg of the chair. Each chair requires four tennis balls.

Consumer Information

Durability	Tennis balls have lasted two to three years in a classroom before losing their effectiveness.
Sound reduction	Sound from chairs moving is reduced to a minimum.
Price	Varies with source.
Color	Ranges from fluorescent yellow to pink.

Where to obtain: One company in Mississauga, Ontario, sells precut tennis balls (called hush-ups) specifically for this purpose. Some teachers have

Reprinted by permission of Carolyn Edwards, MClSC, Auditory Management Services, 83 Watson Avenue, Toronto, Ontario, Canada.

approached local tennis clubs for donations of used tennis balls. Of course, there are always the tennis balls from the roof of the school. Some teachers have put a box at the front of the school for donations from students and staff. Finally, some communities now include tennis balls as an item for recycling.

Teacher comments: When teachers on the second floor have used the tennis balls on chair legs, the teacher underneath on the first floor has been delighted with the reduction in noise. Paradoxically, the elimination of noise has made the children more aware of noise and communication has been easier in the classroom.

Children's comments: Children don't want to remove the tennis balls once the balls have been installed. They say it is easier to hear other children and easier to pay attention in the classroom.

Try hush-ups—one of the easiest improvements to the learning environment!

CHAPTER 10

Measuring Efficacy of Sound Field Placement

Brian M. Kreisman, PhD
Carl C. Crandell, PhD
Joseph J. Smaldino, PhD
Nicole V. Kreisman, MA

KEY POINTS

- Inappropriate classroom acoustics can compromise academic, psychosocial, and psychoeducational performance in children. Whenever modifications are made in the classroom, it is important that the efficacy of those procedures is measured.
- A number of different approaches such as the use of educational performance measures, acoustic measures, objective/subjective speech-perception measures, and functional assessments have been used to document the effects of acoustic interventions and sound field technology on speech recognition, listening, and learning in the classroom.
- Even though one of the most common procedures for measuring the efficacy of acoustical interventions has been to examine global changes in educational achievement through standardized and nonstandardized testing, these measures are difficult to use in establishing unambiguous cause-and-effect relationships in the classroom.
- With functional assessments of efficacy, the teacher, student, or parent completes questionnaires before and after sound field placement. Examples of such assessments include SIFTER, LIFE, SES, and CES.
- Efficacy can also be measured in the classroom with a variety of speech-perception measures (syllables, words, and sentences); however, the

linkage among speech perception, listening, and learning is not well established.

- Efficacy can also be measured via acoustic formulae that have been developed to estimate speech recognition in rooms of varying acoustic qualities. These acoustic formulae include Alcons, AI, STI, RASTI, Direct-to-Reverberant Ratios, and Useful-to-Detrimental Sound Ratios.

This book has amply demonstrated that inappropriate classroom acoustics can compromise academic, psychosocial, and psychoeducational performance in children. Therefore, it is imperative that children be provided an appropriate acoustical environment through acoustical modifications of the classroom environment or placement of sound field technologies. However, whenever modifications are made in the classroom, it is equally important to measure the efficacy of those procedures. Unfortunately, although it is well recognized that such acoustic modifications can benefit speech perception and academic achievement, the efficacy of such procedures is not often measured. Crandell and Smaldino (2000, 2001), for example, reported that less than 20% of audiologists measure efficacy after sound field technology placement. This chapter examines various objective and subjective methodological procedures to assess the efficacy of classroom acoustical modifications and sound field technologies and discusses the following specific areas of efficacy: (1) educational performance measures, (2) acoustic measures, (3) objective and subjective speech-perception measures, and (4) functional assessments.

EFFICACY DEFINED

Efficacy refers to the extrinsic and intrinsic value of the change or modification. Regardless of how acoustic improvements are attempted, whether through physical modifications or the use of assistive technology, a measurable outcome is required in order to prove that the intervention was efficacious. Conversely, outcome measures also can show that the intervention was not effective and that a different modification may be more appropriate. Classrooms are difficult environments in which to conduct such measures. Not only are teachers often reluctant to conduct intrusive and lengthy test procedures, but measures often must be conducted during the school day with all of the students occupying the classroom. The logistics can frequently be intimidating. In spite of such difficulties, a number of different approaches have been used to document the effects of acoustic interventions and sound field technology on speech recognition, listening, and learning in the classroom.

MEASURING EFFICACY THROUGH
EDUCATIONAL PERFORMANCE

One of the most common procedures for measuring the efficacy of acoustical interventions or sound field placement has been to examine global changes in educational achievement, such as standardized and nonstandardized test scores. While such measures intuitively possess high validity, in reality they are often neither valid nor reliable. Specifically, because these measures are so global in nature and are influenced by numerous factors unrelated to the acoustic interventions, using them to establish unambiguous cause-and-effect relationships in the classroom is difficult. One measure of educational performance that has been widely and effectively used in the classroom is on-task behavior. On-task behavior refers to when a student is paying attention to or participating appropriately in the designated classroom activity. Conversely, off-task behavior refers to when the student is not engaged in the designated activity. Off-task behavior is typically evaluated by using functional assessment techniques wherein student behaviors are directly observed during designated classroom activities and tabulated. The tabulation can be used to document off-task behavior and also the antecedents or reasons for the off-task behavior. Indirect functional assessments such as teacher questionnaires or interviews can also provide evidence of off-task behavior. For a detailed discussion concerning procedures to measure on- and off-task behaviors, see Cangelosi (2004).

MEASURING EFFICACY THROUGH
ACOUSTICAL MEASUREMENTS

Acoustical measurements, conducted before and after modifications, are another way to measure the efficacy of classroom interventions. A detailed description of such measurement procedures is found elsewhere in Chapter 6. While the importance of conducting postintervention acoustical measurements is vital and should always be conducted, these procedures do not directly provide data on academic or perceptual benefit. Stated otherwise, although it is reasonable to assume that the reduction of noise and reverberation will improve academic performance, these improvements need to be measured in a more direct manner.

MEASURING EFFICACY THROUGH
FUNCTIONAL ASSESSMENTS

With functional assessments of efficacy, the teacher, student, or parent completes a questionnaire, or questionnaires, before and after sound field placement. There are a number of functional assessments of efficacy that are commercially available. Perhaps the most widely used of these questionnaires is the Screening Instrument for Targeting Educational Risk (SIFTER) (Anderson, 1989). The SIFTER allows the teacher to observe and rate each student (or classroom of students) in five content areas: academics, attention, communication, class participation, and school behavior. The total score in each content area is then categorized as pass, marginal, or fail. A preschool version of the SIFTER was developed to evaluate younger children (three years of age through kindergarten) (Anderson & Matkin, 1996). While originally intended as a tool to help identify students at risk for listening problems, it has proven to be useful in establishing efficacy of intervention in the classroom. When used in a pretest-posttest experimental design, any change in student performance as a result of classroom acoustic intervention can be documented. It should be noted that there is also a preschool version of the SIFTER available. An extension of the SIFTER called the Listening Inventories for Education (LIFE) (Anderson & Smaldino, 1998) retains a teacher self-report questionnaire but also adds a self-report questionnaire that is completed by the student. By obtaining direct input from the student regarding listening difficulties in the classroom, the overall validity of the subjective approach to efficacy should be improved.

The Children's Auditory Performance Scale (CHAPS) is another questionnaire that can be used to quantify the observed auditory behaviors of children. The questionnaire can be used for children seven years of age and older. The CHAPS is a questionnaire-type scale consisting of thirty-six items concerning six listening conditions or functions (subsections): (1) quiet, (2) ideal, (3) multiple inputs, (4) noise, (5) auditory memory/sequencing, and (6) auditory attention span. These six subsections were chosen to represent the most often reported auditory difficulties of children diagnosed as having an auditory processing disorder (APD). Respondents, usually parents or teachers, are asked to judge the amount of listening difficulty experienced by a child compared to the listening difficulty of a child of similar age and background.

Crandell, Smaldino, and Kreisman (2004) recently developed the Classroom Acoustical Modification Efficacy Scale (CES), the Frequency Modulation (FM) Efficacy Scale (FES), and the Sound Field Efficacy Scale (SES). The CES, FES, and SES use an open-ended format that allows the teacher to list, in order of importance, specific listening or learning needs prior to classroom modification. The teacher then indicates the degree of change, if any, in the previously stated areas of need following the classroom modifications. The scales are unique in that they may provide for individualized teacher input regarding the needs of the particular classroom, which encourages teacher engagement and investment in the modification process. Samples of these scales are located in Appendix 10-A.

MEASURING EFFICACY THROUGH
BEHAVIORAL SPEECH-PERCEPTION TESTS

Efficacy can also be measured in the classroom with a variety of speech-perception measures (syllables, words, and sentences). Each of these speech-perception tests can provide the investigator with different and pertinent aspects of the perceptual effects of the classroom treatment. For example, tests such as the Modified Rhyme Test that allow for consonant confusion analyses may allow researchers to pinpoint specific problems not only with the acoustics of the room, but also with perceptual differences between students in the classroom. In contrast to syllabic stimuli, tests using word and sentence stimuli may provide more real-world contextual information regarding perceptual processes due to their higher linguistic content. While speech-perception materials are intuitively pleasing, the linkage among speech perception, listening, and learning is not well established. In addition, speech-perception testing may be difficult to conduct in the classroom due to the length or complexity of the test protocols.

MEASURING EFFICACY THROUGH ACOUSTICAL FORMULAE

Efficacy can also be measured via acoustic formulae that have been developed to estimate speech recognition in rooms of varying acoustic qualities. Unfortunately, most of these indices were developed for adult listeners with normal hearing and may not be applicable for children, particularly children with sensorineural hearing loss (SNHL). Moreover, such procedures require the use of specialized equipment that may not be readily accessible to many readers. Examples of such formulae are provided below.

Articulation Loss of Consonants (Alcons)

The Articulation Loss of Consonants (Alcons) (Peutz, 1971) expresses the percent loss of consonant definition. The percentage of lost consonants for listeners within the critical distance can be calculated as

$$Alcons = \left(\frac{M200D^2T^2}{V} = a \right)\%$$ (10.1)

and for listeners beyond the critical distance as

$$Alcons = (9T = a)\%1$$ (10.2)

where D = distance from the speaker to the listener (in meters), T = reverberation time (at 1,400 Hz), V = volume of the room in cubic meters, and a = zero correction (constant for a good listener, which varies between 1.5% and 12.5% for different listeners within the listening group). A high Alcons value indicates a greater loss of intelligibility. Measurements for the Alcons are based on a single one-third-octave band centered at 2,000 Hz and do not account for many factors, such as reverberation, that can dramatically reduce speech intelligibility. Therefore, the Alcons often overestimates the intelligibility scores that would actually be obtained in reverberant environments.

Articulation Index (AI)

The Articulation Index (AI) (French & Steinberg, 1947) is a prediction of the perception of transmitted or processed speech. To compute the AI, the speech frequencies are divided into twenty frequency bands, usually one-third-octave bands. Each band is assumed to contribute independently to the overall intelligibility. The S/N ratio is computed for each band, then weighted and combined to yield the AI. Specifically, the articulation index is calculated as

$$AI = \sum_{1}^{n} W \cdot \Delta A_m, \tag{10.3}$$

where n = number of bands, ΔA_m = the maximum value of the S/N ratio, and W = the fractional part of ΔA_m, which is contributed by a band with a particular S/N ratio. The AI is expressed as a number between 0 and 1, where an AI of 0 predicts that speech is unintelligible and an AI of 1 predicts that speech is completely intelligible.

Speech Transmission Index (STI)

The Speech Transmission Index (STI) (Houtgast, Steeneken, & Plomp, 1980) is a measure of speech intelligibility based on modulation transfer function (MTF) theory. The MTF is a function of modulation frequency that reflects the effect of the room (noise and reverberation) on the modulation index of a (hypothetical) test signal. The MTF function, $m(F)$, can be defined as

$$m(F) = \left[1 = \left(2\pi F \frac{T}{13.8}\right)^2\right]^{-1/2} \left[1 + 10^{(-S/N)/10}\right]^{-1} \tag{10.4}$$

where F = frequency and T = reverberation time. The $m(F)$ function is calculated for each of the eighteen one-third-octave intervals. The eighteen $m(F)$ values are converted into eighteen apparent SNRs after each $m(F)$ is clipped when exceeding the range of ±15 dB. Hence, the STI is calculated as

$$STI = \frac{[\overline{(S/N)}_{app} + 15]}{30} \tag{10.5}$$

where $\overline{(S/N)}_{app}$ = the mean apparent SNR. The STI values vary from 0 to 1. An STI of 0 predicts that speech is unintelligible, and an STI of 1.0 predicts that speech is completely intelligible. A special test signal that has characteristics similar to speech is utilized in STI testing. The STI follows the concept that speech is composed of two spectra: the audible spectrum (the speech we hear) and the modulation spectrum (the frequency of phoneme production). The modulation spectrum can be represented by fourteen one-third-octave intervals from 0.4 to about 20 Hz. The depth of the modulation of the received signal is compared with that of the transmitted signal within each band. A reduction in the modulation depth is associated with a loss of intelligibility.

Rapid Speech Transmission Index (RASTI)

The Rapid Speech Transmission Index (RASTI) (Houtgast & Steeneken, 1984) was developed as a simpler alternative to the more complex STI. Similar to the STI, RASTI values vary from 0 to 1, where 0 predicts that speech is completely unintelligible and 1 predicts that speech is completely intelligible. Likewise, RASTI uses a speechlike signal and correlates reductions in modulation depth to loss of intelligibility. Unlike the STI, however, RASTI uses only two octave bands, one centered at 500 Hz and the other centered at 2,000 Hz. The calculation for RASTI is

$$RASTI = \frac{[(\overline{S/N})_{app} + 15]}{30} \tag{10.6}$$

where $(\overline{S/N})_{app}$ = the mean apparent SNR.

Direct-to-Reverberant Ratios

The quantities C_{50} and C_{80} express speech clarity as ratios between the intensity of the direct sound and the intensity of the reverberant sound (Bradley, 1986). Specifically, C_{50} measures the energy ratio of the first 50 milliseconds (ms) of direct sound to the overall steady-state reverberation, whereas C_{80} measures the first 80 ms. The formula to calculate clarity is

$$C = \log \int_0^{80ms} p^2 dt \bigg/ \int_{80ms}^{\infty} p^2 dt \tag{10.7}$$

The speech clarity ratio is expressed in decibels, ranging from –30 dB to +30 dB, with a minimum acceptable value of 0 dB and a preferred value of at least +4 dB.

Useful-to-Detrimental Sound Ratios

The useful-to-detrimental sound ratios express the ratio, in dB, between sounds that are useful to intelligibility and sounds that are detrimental to it. Lochner and Burger (1964) suggested that early reflected sound within the first 95 ms increased speech perception (i.e., useful) whereas the reflected sound arriving after the first 95 ms reduced speech perception (i.e., detrimental). The useful-to-detrimental ratio U_{95} can be expressed as

$$R_{sn} = 101 \log \frac{\int_0^{95} \alpha P^2 \, dt}{\int_{95}^{\infty} P^2 \, dt = P_n^2 \Delta t} \text{ dB,} \qquad (10.8)$$

where α = a fraction of the reflected energy relative to the direct sound (for different levels and delay times), P = the instantaneous value of the sound pressure due to the pulse, P_n = a root mean square (rms) pressure, t = time in ms, and Δt = the duration of the pulse used for measurement. The U_{50} and U_{80} ratios are more commonly used today. Speech sounds are "useful" when they arrive within the first 50 or 80 ms after the direct sound. These sounds are perceptually integrated with the direct sound. "Detrimental" sounds are determined by adding the speech energy arriving later than 50 or 80 ms and the ambient noise in the room. For example, the U_{50} ratio, in decibels, can be described as

$$U_{50} = 10 \log \left(\frac{E_d + E_e}{E_l + E_n} \right) \qquad (10.9)$$

where E_d = the direct energy from the speaker, E_e = the early arriving reflected energy from the speaker, E_l = the late arriving reflected energy, and E_n = noise energy.

SUMMARY

Whenever sound field technology is utilized in a classroom, it is vital to measure efficacy to verify the effectiveness of that intervention. Unfortunately, no single methodology provides all of the perceptual and academic information necessary. Consequently, it is strongly recommended that a multifaceted and multidisciplinary approach to measuring efficacy be used. Such an approach should include as many of the above-mentioned procedures as possible and would incorporate such disciplines as audiology, architecture, and acoustical engineering.

DISCUSSION TOPICS

1. Discuss why conducting efficacy measures is vital after acoustical modifications or sound field placement are utilized in the classroom.
2. Describe the advantages and disadvantages of using educational performance in measuring the efficacy of acoustical modifications or sound field placement.

3. Describe the advantages and disadvantages of using speech-perception tests in measuring the efficacy of acoustical modifications or sound field placement.
4. Describe the advantages and disadvantages of using objective measurements in measuring the efficacy of acoustical modifications or sound field placement.
5. Describe the advantages and disadvantages of using functional questionnaires in measuring the efficacy of acoustical modifications or sound field placement.

REFERENCES

Anderson, K. (1989). *Screening instrument for targeting educational risk (SIFTER)*. Tampa, FL: Educational Audiology Association.

Anderson, K., & Matkin, N. (1996). *The preschool screening instrument for targeting educational risk*. Tampa, FL: Educational Audiology Association.

Anderson, K., & Smaldino, J. (1998). *The listening inventories for education (LIFE)*. Tampa, FL: Educational Audiology Association.

Bradley, J. (1986). Speech intelligibility studies in classrooms. *Journal of the Acoustical Society of America, 80*(3), 846–854.

Cangelosi, J. (2004). *Classroom management strategies gaining and maintaining students' cooperation* (5th ed.). New York: Longman.

Crandell, C., & Smaldino, J. (2000). Room acoustics for listeners with normal hearing and hearing impairment. In M. Valente, R. Roeser, & H. Hosford-Dunn (Eds.), *Audiology: Treatment strategies* (pp. 601–637). New York: Thieme Medical Publishers.

Crandell, C., & Smaldino, J. (2001). Auditory rehabilitation technology and room acoustics. In J. Katz (Ed.), *Handbook of audiology* (pp. 654–675). New York: Williams & Wilkins.

Crandell, C., Smaldino, J., & Kreisman, B. (2004). *CES, FES, & SES: Efficacy scales for classrooms*. Gainesville, FL: The Listening Source.

French, N., & Steinberg, J. (1947). Factors governing the intelligibility of speech sounds. *Journal of the Acoustical Society of America, 19*, 90–91.

Houtgast, T., & Steeneken, H. (1984). A multi-language evaluation of the RASTI method or estimating speech intelligibility in auditoria. *Acustica, 54*, 185–199.

Houtgast, T., Steeneken, H. J. M., & Plomp, R. (1980). Predicting speech intelligibility in rooms from the modulation transfer function. *Acustica, 46*, 60–72.

Lochner, J., & Burger, J. (1964). The influence of reflections in auditorium acoustics. *Journal of Sound Vibration, 4*, 426–454.

Peutz, V. (1971). Articulation loss of consonants as a criterion for speech transmission in a room. *Journal of the Audio Engineering Society, 19*, 915–919.

APPENDIX 10-A
EFFICACY FORMS

- SIFTER: Screening Instrument for Targeting Educational Risk
- Preschool SIFTER: Screening Instrument for Targeting Educational Risk in Preschool Children (Age 3–Kindergarten)
- LIFE: Listening Inventory for Education: Teacher Appraisal of Listening Difficulty
- LIFE: Listening Inventory for Education: Student Appraisal of Listening Difficulty
- CHAPS: Children's Auditory Performance Scale
- Classroom Acoustical Modification Efficacy Scale (CES-1)
- FM Amplification Efficacy Scale I (FES-1)
- Sound Field Amplification Efficacy Scale I (SES-1)

S.I.F.T.E.R.

SCREENING INSTRUMENT FOR TARGETING EDUCATIONAL RISK
by Karen L. Anderson, Ed.S., CCC-A

STUDENT _____ TEACHER _____ GRADE _____

DATE COMPLETED _____ SCHOOL _____ DISTRICT _____

The above child is suspect for hearing problems which may or may not be affecting his/her school performance. This rating scale has been designed to sift out students who are educationally at risk possibly as a result of hearing problems.

Based on your knowledge from observations of this student, circle the number best representing his/her behavior. After answering the questions, please record any comments about the student in the space provided on the reverse side.

1. What is your estimate of the student's class standing in comparison of that of his/her classmates?	UPPER 5	4	MIDDLE 3	2	LOWER 1		ACADEMICS
2. How does the student's achievement compare to your estimation of her/his potential?	EQUAL 5	4	LOWER 3	2	MUCH LOWER 1		
3. What is the student's reading level, reading ability group or reading readiness group in the classroom (e.g., a student with average reading ability performs in the middle group)?	UPPER 5	4	MIDDLE 3	2	LOWER 1		
4. How distractible is the student in comparison to his/her classmates?	NOT VERY 5	4	AVERAGE 3	2	VERY 1		ATTENTION
5. What is the student's attention span in comparison to that of his/her classmates?	LONGER 5	4	AVERAGE 3	2	SHORTER 1		
6. How often does the student hesitate or become confused when responding to oral directions (e.g., "Turn to page . . .")?	NEVER 5		OCCASIONALLY 3		FREQUENTLY 1		
7. How does the student's comprehension compare to the average understanding ability of her/his classmates?	ABOVE 5	4	AVERAGE 3	2	BELOW 1		COMMUNICATION
8. How does the student's vocabulary and word usage skills compare with those of other students in his/her age group?	ABOVE 5	4	AVERAGE 3	2	BELOW 1		
9. How proficient is the student at telling a story or relating happenings from home when compared to classmates?	ABOVE 5	4	AVERAGE 3	2	BELOW 1		
10. How often does the student volunteer information to class discussions or in answer to teacher questions?	FREQUENTLY 5	4	OCCASIONALLY 3	2	NEVER 1		CLASS PARTICIPATION
11. With what frequency does the student complete his/her class and homework assignments within the time allocated?	ALWAYS 5	4	USUALLY 3	2	SELDOM 1		
12. After instruction, does the student have difficulty starting to work (looks at other students working or asks for help)?	NEVER 5	4	OCCASIONALLY 3	2	FREQUENTLY 1		
13. Does the student demonstrate any behaviors that seem unusual or inappropriate when compared to other students?	NEVER 5	4	OCCASIONALLY 3	2	FREQUENTLY 1		SCHOOL BEHAVIOR
14. Does the student become frustrated easily, sometimes to the point of losing emotional control?	NEVER 5	4	OCCASIONALLY 3	2	FREQUENTLY 1		
15. In general, how would you rank the student's relationship with peers (ability to get along with others)?	GOOD 5	4	AVERAGE 3	2	POOR 1		

202

(form continued from previous page)

TEACHER COMMENTS

Has this child repeated a grade, had frequent absences or experienced health problems (including ear infections and colds)? Has the student received, or is he/she now receiving, special support services? Does the child have any other health problems that may be pertinent to his/her educational functioning?

The S.I.F.T.E.R. is a SCREENING TOOL ONLY

Any student failing this screening in a content area as determined on the scoring grid below should be considered for further assessment, depending on his/her individual needs as per school district criteria. For example, failing in the Academics area suggests an educational assessment, in the Communication area a speech-language assessment, and in the School Behavior area an assessment by a psychologist or a social worker. Failing in the Attention and/or Class Participation area in combination with other areas may suggest an evaluation by an educational audiologist. Children placed in the marginal area are at risk for failing and should be monitored or considered for assessment depending upon additional information.

SCORING

Sum the responses to the three questions in each content area and record in the appropriate box on the reverse side and under Total Score below. Place an **X** on the number that corresponds most closely with the content area score (e.g., if a teacher circled 3, 4 and 2 for the questions in the Academics area, an **X** would be placed on the number 9 across from the Academics content area). Connect the **X**'s to make a profile.

CONTENT AREA	TOTAL SCORE	PASS						MARGINAL		FAIL				
ACADEMICS		15	14	13	12	11	10	9	8	7	6	5	4	3
ATTENTION		15	14	13	12	11	10	9	8	7	6	5	4	3
COMMUNICATION		15	14	13	12	11		10	9 8	7	6	5	4	3
CLASS PARTICIPATION		15	14	13	12	11	10	9	8 7	6	5	4	3	
SOCIAL BEHAVIOR		15	14	13	12	11	10	9	8	7	6	5	4	3

PRESCHOOL S.I.F.T.E.R.

Screening Instrument for Targeting Educational Risk
in Preschool Children (age 3-Kindergarten)
by Karen L. Anderson, Ed.S. & Noel Matkin, Ph.D.

Child ——————————————————— Teacher ——————————— Age ————

Date Completed ____/____/____ School ——————————————————— District ————

The above child is suspect for hearing problems which may affect his/her ability to listen, pay attention, develop language, follow teacher instruction and learn normally. This rating scale has been designed to sift out children who are at risk for educational delay and who may need further evaluation. Based on your knowledge of this child, circle the number that best represents his/her behavior. If the child is a member of a class that has students with special needs, comparisons should be made to normal learning classmates or normal developmental milestones. Please share additional comments about the child on the reverse side of this form.

1. How well does the child understand basic concepts when compared to classmates (e.g., colors, shapes, etc.)?	ABOVE 5	AVERAGE 4　　3	BELOW 2　　1	PREACADEMICS
2. How often is the child able to follow two-part directions?	ALWAYS 5	FREQUENTLY 4　　3	SELDOM 2　　1	
3. How well does the child participate in group activities when compared to classmates (e.g., calendar, sharing)?	ABOVE 5	AVERAGE 4　　3	BELOW 2　　1	
4. How distractible is the child in comparison to his/her classmates during large group activities?	SELDOM 5	OCCASIONAL 4　　3	FREQUENT 2　　1	ATTENTION
5. What is the child's attention span in comparison to classmates?	LONGER 5	AVERAGE 4　　3	SHORTER 2　　1	
6. How well does the child pay attention during a small group activity or story time?	ABOVE 5	AVERAGE 4　　3	BELOW 2　　1	
7. How does the child's vocabulary and word usage skills compare to classmates?	ABOVE 5	AVERAGE 4　　3	BELOW 2　　1	COMMUNICATION
8. How proficient is the child at relating an event when compared to classmates?	ABOVE 5	AVERAGE 4　　3	BELOW 2　　1	
9. How does the child's overall speech intelligibility compare to classmates (i.e., production of speech sounds)?	ABOVE 5	AVERAGE 4　　3	BELOW 2　　1	
10. How often does the child answer questions appropriately (verbal or signed)?	ALMOST ALWAYS 5	FREQUENTLY 4　　3	SELDOM 2　　1	CLASS PARTICIPATION
11. How often does the child share information during group discussions?	ALMOST ALWAYS 5	FREQUENTLY 4　　3	SELDOM 2　　1	
12. How often does the child participate with classmates in group activities or group play?	ALMOST ALWAYS 5	FREQUENTLY 4　　3	SELDOM 2　　1	
13. Does the child play in socially acceptable ways (i.e., turn taking, sharing)?	ALMOST ALWAYS 5	FREQUENTLY 4　　3	SELDOM 2　　1	SOCIAL BEHAVIOR
14. How proficient is the child at using verbal language or sign language to communicate effectively with classmates (e.g., asking to play with another child's toy)?	ABOVE 5	AVERAGE 4　　3	BELOW 2　　1	
15. How often does the child become frustrated, sometimes to the point of losing emotional control?	NEVER 5	SELDOM 4　　3	FREQUENTLY 2　　1	

(form continued from previous page)

TEACHER COMMENTS: (frequent absences, health problems, other problems or handicaps in addition to hearing?)

The Preschool S.I.F.T.E.R. is a SCREENING TOOL ONLY. The primary goal of the Preschool S.I.F.T.E.R. is to identify those children who are at-risk for developmental or educational problems due to hearing problems and who merit further observation and investigation. Analysis has revealed that two factors, expressive communication and socially appropriate behavior, discriminate children who are normal from those who are at-risk. The greater the degree of hearing problem, the greater the impact on these two factors and the higher the validity of this screening measure. If a child is found to be at-risk then the examiner is encouraged to calculate the total score in each of the five content areas. Analysis of the content area score may assist in developing a profile of the child's strengths and special needs. The profile may prove beneficial in determining appropriate areas for evaluation and developing an individual program for the child.

SCORING
There are two steps to the scoring process. First, enter scores for each of the indicated questions in the spaces provided and sum the total of the 6 questions for the expressive communication factor and then the 4 questions for the socially appropriate behavior factor. If the child's scores fall into the At-Risk category for either or both of these factors, then sum the 3 questions in each content area to develop a profile of the child's strengths and potential areas of need.

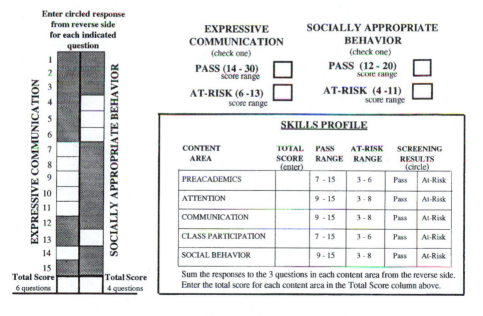

CONTENT AREA	TOTAL SCORE (enter)	PASS RANGE	AT-RISK RANGE	SCREENING RESULTS (circle)	
PREACADEMICS		7 - 15	3 - 6	Pass	At-Risk
ATTENTION		9 - 15	3 - 8	Pass	At-Risk
COMMUNICATION		9 - 15	3 - 8	Pass	At-Risk
CLASS PARTICIPATION		7 - 15	3 - 6	Pass	At-Risk
SOCIAL BEHAVIOR		9 - 15	3 - 8	Pass	At-Risk

Sum the responses to the 3 questions in each content area from the reverse side. Enter the total score for each content area in the Total Score column above.

L.I.F.E.

Listening Inventory For Education
An Efficacy Tool
Teacher Appraisal of Listening Difficulty
By Karen L. Anderson, Ed.S. & Joseph J. Smaldino, Ph.D.

Name_____ Grade_____ Date_____

School_____ Teacher_____

Hearing Aid User Y / N   Trial Period   Type of Classroom

Trial Period   Y / N   Length___Weeks   Hearing Technology_____

Instructions: Circle the item which best describes the student's listening and learning behaviors.
See reverse for suggestions to aid this student in listening and understanding classroom instruction.

The student's:

	AGREE	NO CHANGE	Not Observed	DISAGREE	
1. Focus on instruction has improved (more tuned in to instruction).	(2)	(1)	(0)	(-1)	(-2)
2. Appears to understand class instruction better.	(2)	(1)	(0)	(-1)	(-2)
3. Overall attention span has improved (less fidgety and/or less distracted).	(2)	(1)	(0)	(-1)	(-2)
4. Attention has improved when listening to directions presented to whole class.	(2)	(1)	(0)	(-1)	(-2)
5. Stays on task longer with less need for redirection.	(2)	(1)	(0)	(-1)	(-2)
6. Follows directions more quickly or easily (less hesitation before beginning work).	(2)	(1)	(0)	(-1)	(-2)
7. Answers questions in a more appropriate way or answers appropriately more often.	(2)	(1)	(0)	(-1)	(-2)
8. Improved understanding of instructional videos and/or morning announcements.	(2)	(1)	(0)	(-1)	(-2)
9. More involved in class discussions (volunteers more often, follows better).	(2)	(1)	(0)	(-1)	(-2)
10. Improved understanding of answers or comments by peers during discussions.	(2)	(1)	(0)	(-1)	(-2)
11. Improved attention and understanding when background noise is present (ie., transitions).	(2)	(1)	(0)	(-1)	(-2)
12. Improved ability to discriminate auditorilly (understand similar words or sounds).	(2)	(1)	(0)	(-1)	(-2)
13. Attention improved when listening in groups (small group/cooperative learning activities).	(2)	(1)	(0)	(-1)	(-2)
14. Socially involved more with other children or more comfortable in peer conversations.	(2)	(1)	(0)	(-1)	(-2)
15. Rate of learning seems to have improved (quicker to comprehend instruction).	(2)	(1)	(0)	(-1)	(-2)
16. Based on my knowledge and observations I believe that the amplification system is beneficial to the student's overall attention, listening and learning in the classroom.	(5)	(2)	(0)	(-2)	(-5)

Comments: (e.g., absences, equipment use problems)

Total Appraisal Score _____

Place an X on the continuum below to record the appraisal score:

Strong support for Positive Change: Use is Highly Beneficial	Support for Positive Change: Use is Beneficial	No Change: Benefit of Use Not Identified	Support for Negative Change: Use is Unfavorable	Strong support for Negative Change: Use is Highly Unfavorable
35 · · · · · · · · · · ·	· 17 · · · · · · · · · · ·	0 · · · · · · · · · ·	· -17 · · · · · · · · ·	-35

LISTENING INVENTORY FOR EDUCATION
SUGGESTIONS FOR ACCOMMODATING STUDENTS WITH AUDITORY DIFFICULTIES

Students with auditory problems face extra challenges learning in a typical classroom setting. Typically, they can hear the teacher talk, but miss parts of speech or do not hear clearly, especially if noise is present. Students usually do not know what they didn't hear because they didn't hear it. They often may not know that they "misheard" a message unless they have already had experience with the language and topic under discussion. Use of amplification, having fluctuating hearing ability, hearing loss in just one ear, permanent hearing loss of any degree or central auditory processing disorders all compromise a student's ability to focus on verbal instruction and comprehend the fragments of speech information that are heard. The following items are suggestions for accomodating these student's special auditory needs and helping them learn their best in your classroom.

1. Seat the student close to where you customarily teach.
Sound weakens as it crosses distance. If a student has any auditory difficulties, how close you are to him/her will make a big difference on how well the student can hear and understand you.
- Can the student be moved to the front of the room?
- Can the student be allowed flexible seating so they can move to a better vantage point as classroom activities change? (e.g. move close to TV during movies)
- If your teaching style causes you to move around the room when you talk, is it possible to stay in close proximity to the student with auditory problems?
- When giving test directions, can you see the student's face clearly? Are you standing near the student's desk? Is the lighting on your face and not from a window behind you? Be sure the student is watching you.
- Develop a signal the student can use if he or she does not understand or has missed critical information.

2. Be aware of the benefits and limitations of lipreading.
- Only about 30-40% of speech sounds are visible on the lips. Lipreading supplements a student's hearing but is most helpful when the topic of conversation and vocabulary are known. New concepts and new vocabulary words have little meaning using lipreading.
- Is the student seated so they can see your face clearly? Too close and they view your face from a skewed angle, too far and the quick, tiny mouth movements are imperceptible.
- Lipreading is only possible if you are facing the student. If you use the chalkboard, do not provide verbal instruction while writing or be prepared to summarize or repeat that information for the student.
- Reading aloud to the class with your face downward makes lipreading very difficult. Hold the book below your chin so your face is easily visualized.
- Students cannot lipread and take notes at the same time. Classroom notetakers can use carbonized (NCR) paper and share notes easily. The student can use these notes from other students to fill in gaps in understanding.
- The extra demands of trying to understand using only speech fragments and of constantly trying to lipread can be very fatiguing. Listening breaks are natural, especially after rapid class discussions, lectures or new information.

3. Noise is a barrier to learning.
- Adults and children with normal hearing usually can tolerate a small amount of background noise without having their speech understanding compromised. Students with auditory problems are already missing fragments of what is said, especially if a message is spoken farther than from 3-6 feet away. Noise covers up word endings and brief words, reverberation smears the word fragments that are perceived.
- Can the student be allowed flexible seating so they can move away from noise sources? (e.g. lawn mower)
- Overhead projectors allow the student to clearly view the teacher's face, however, their fan noise interferes with understanding. If the student has a poorer hearing ear, face that one toward the overhead projector (or noisy ventilator, etc.) and seat close, but not next to the projector.
- If possible, eliminate or dampen unnecessary noise sources. Sometimes apsorbtive material, such as styrofoam or a thick bathtowel placed under an aquarium heater or animal cage will absorb some noise. Seat the student away from animal distractions.
- Keep your classroom door closed, especially when classes pass in the hall, gym or lunchroom activities are audible.
- One of the main causes of noise in the classroom is due to the activity of students. Seat away from peers who are very active or habitually noisy. Allow student's time to search their desks so that the noise generated will not occur during verbal instruction. Inform the custodian of especially squeaky desks.

4. Control or allow for distance.
- During group discussion, students with auditory problems typically can understand the students seated next to them but cannot understand students who are answering from more distant seats.
- Use a student's name when calling on them to answer a question. This will allow the student with hearing needs a chance to turn to face the answering student and to lipread if at all possible.
- Summarize key points given by classmates, especially brief messages like numeric answers, yes/no, etc.
- Allow or assign a student buddy that the student with auditory problems can ask for clarification or cueing.

207

L. I. F. E.

Listening Inventory For Education
An Efficacy Tool
Student Appraisal of Listening Difficulty

By Karen L. Anderson, Ed.S. & Joseph J. Smaldino, Ph.D.

Post-test Date_____

Name_____ Grade_____ Pretest Date_____
Can also be used for evaluating trial periods of sound field amplification use for all students in a classroom.

School_____ Teacher_____
Hearing Aid User Y / N   Trial Period   Type of Classroom
Trial Period Y / N   Length____Weeks   Hearing Technology_____

Instructions: Circle the item which best describes the student's difficulty listening in the situations shown on picture card items 1-10. Optional items 11-16 can be scored if these situations are encountered in the school environment. See reverse for intervention suggestions to improve class listening and understanding.

Classroom Listening Situations	ALWAYS EASY	MOSTLY EASY	SOMETIMES DIFFICULT	MOSTLY DIFFICULT	ALWAYS DIFFICULT
1. Teacher talking in front of room Comments:	(10)	(7)	(5)	(2)	(0)
2. Teacher talking during transition time Comments:	(10)	(7)	(5)	(2)	(0)
3. Teacher talking with back turned Comments:	(10)	(7)	(5)	(2)	(0)
4. Listening with hallway noise present Comments:	(10)	(7)	(5)	(2)	(0)
5. Other students making noise Comments:	(10)	(7)	(5)	(2)	(0)
6. Student answering during discussion Comments:	(10)	(7)	(5)	(2)	(0)
7. Listening with overhead projector fan on Comments:	(10)	(7)	(5)	(2)	(0)
8. Teacher talking while moving Comments:	(10)	(7)	(5)	(2)	(0)
9. Word recognition during a test or directions Comments:	(10)	(7)	(5)	(2)	(0)
10. Simultaneous large and small group Comments:	(10)	(7)	(5)	(2)	(0)

Additional Listening Situations

	ALWAYS EASY	MOSTLY EASY	SOMETIMES DIFFICULT	MOSTLY DIFFICULT	ALWAYS DIFFICULT
11. Cooperative small group learning	(20)	(15)	(10)	(5)	(0)
12. Listening in gym (inside & outside)	(20)	(15)	(10)	(5)	(0)
13. Listening in school assembly	(20)	(15)	(10)	(5)	(0)
14. Listening to students during lunch	(20)	(15)	(10)	(5)	(0)
15. Students talking while coats are hung up	(20)	(15)	(10)	(5)	(0)

Scoring   PRE-TEST   POST-TEST
Sum of Items 1 - 10   (100 possible) _____ CLASSROOM LISTENING SCORE _____
Sum of Items 11-16   (100 possible) _____ ADDITIONAL SITUATIONS SCORE _____

The LIFE Student Appraisal was inspired by the Hearing Performance Inventory for Children. The authors recognize T. Giolas, A. Brancia Maxon & A. Riordan Kessler for their work in developing the HPIC.

LISTENING INVENTORY FOR EDUCATION
SUGGESTIONS FOR IMPROVING CLASSROOM LISTENING

Mark an X next to each statement that corresponds with the situations indicated on the reverse side in which the student is experiencing any difficulty.

Classroom Difficult Listening Situations

__X__ 1. Let the teacher know that you cannot understand. Develop a signal system with your teacher.

__X__ 1. Be sure that you are seated near the teacher. Ask to move if needed.

_____ 2. Ask a student buddy to explain the directions ("Did she say page 191?").

_____ 2. Before the teacher hands out a test to the class, ask what kind of test it is and how you take it (fill in all blanks, true/false, multiple choice).

_____ 3. Have another student or two in your class that will share their class notes with you; the teacher can help to arrange this and provide carbonized paper. It is still your job to listen very carefully as your teacher talks. Notes can help you fill in gaps you may have missed as you study later.

_____ 3. Be sure that the teacher is aware of how important it is for you to see his/her face. Ask your parent to send a note to the teacher. Ask for the teacher to repeat information, ask a neighbor, use your signal.

_____ 4. If there is noise in the hall, ask for door to be closed. Arrange with your teacher ahead of time to have permission to get up and close the door whenever it's noisy.

_____ 5. Let your teacher know that noise from classmates is interfering with your understanding; use your signal system to alert your teacher that it's too noisy.

_____ 6. Ask your teacher to say student's names when calling on them to answer questions. Watch her face and listen carefully for names so you can quickly turn to face the talking student.

_____ 6. If you miss information from student answers or discussion: 1) ask answering student to repeat the information. 2) ask the teacher to repeat, 3) ask a neighbor

_____ 7. If you did not hear all of the announcements, ask the teacher or a neighbor what they were about.

_____ 8. If you cannot understand what the teacher is saying as he or she talks when the class is getting out books or papers it is important to be sure you are ready and watching the teacher during these times. If you miss a page number or other information be sure to raise your hand and ask - you are probably not the only one who didn't hear the teacher clearly in all the noise of changing activities.

_____ 9. Spelling tests are easiest if you really know the word list and can tell the difference between similar words (e.g., champion and trampoline have similar sounds but have different endings). Sit close and watch the teacher's face carefully. If you are not sure you clearly heard a word, let the teacher know immediately (you could use your signal).

_____ 10. Hearing speech clearly in a movie can be hard because of the background music on some videos. Sit close to the TV even if it means sitting in a different seat. If used, ask the teacher to put the FM microphone next to the TV. Have a note taker. Request closed captioned videos be used.

Additional Difficult Listening Situations

_____ 11. In small group work, be sure to sit close to other students and try to be able to see all of their faces. If used, pass the FM microphone from student to student. Ask students to repeat what you missed. It helps if your group could meet in a quieter spot of the class or in the hall while you work.

_____ 12. While in the gym, stand close to the teacher for directions and ask other children for directions you may have missed. Ask the teacher to repeat what you missed. Use a signal system to let your teacher know you didn't understand.

_____ 13. To hear in an assembly it is important to be near the front. If you have a personal FM the person speaking should wear the transmitter.

_____ 14. Ask your friends to repeat or clarify when something is missed (Did you say tomorrow night?"). Sit where you can easily see their faces and try to sit away from noisier children or noisy areas of your classroom. Remind your friends they may need to tap you to get your attention when it's really noisy and if you are not watching their faces.

_____ 15. You need to depend on your friends to catch your eye, tap you or for them to wait until they see you looking at them before they talk to you. Ask them to repeat what you have missed (Practice is at what time? You called Suzy when?).

C. H. A. P. S.

Children's Auditory Performance Scale

by Walter J. Smoski, Ph.D., Michael A. Brunt, Ph.D., J. Curtis Tannahill, Ph.D.

Child's Name_____ Age (years____ months_____) Date Completed_____
Name of Person
Completing CHAPS_____ Relationship to Child _____

PLEASE READ INSTRUCTIONS CAREFULLY

Answer all questions by comparing this child to other children of similar age and background. Do not answer the questions based only on the difficulty of the listening condition. For example, all 8-year-old children, to a certain extent, may not hear and understand when listening in a noisy room; this would be a difficult listening condition for all children. However, some children may have more difficulty in this listening condition than others. You must judge whether or not THIS child has MORE difficulty than other children in each listening condition cited. Please make your judgment using the following response choices. CIRCLE a number for each item. For ages 7 and above.

The response columns are:
LESS DIFFICULT / SAME AMOUNT OF DIFFICULTY / SLIGHTLY MORE DIFFICULT / MORE DIFFICULT / CONSIDERABLY MORE DIFFICULT / SIGNIFICANTLY MORE DIFFICULT / CANNOT FUNCTION AT ALL

LISTENING CONDITION

NOISE

TOTAL CONDITION SCORE [ ]

If listening in a room where there is background noise such as TV, music, others talking, children playing, etc., this child has difficulty hearing and understanding compared to other children of similar age and background

	LESS DIFFICULT	SAME AMOUNT OF DIFFICULTY	SLIGHTLY MORE DIFFICULT	MORE DIFFICULT	CONSIDERABLY MORE DIFFICULT	SIGNIFICANTLY MORE DIFFICULT	CANNOT FUNCTION AT ALL
1. When paying attention	+1	0	-1	-2	-3	-4	-5
2. When being asked a question	+1	0	-1	-2	-3	-4	-5
3. When being given simple instructions	+1	0	-1	-2	-3	-4	-5
4. When being given complicated, multiple instructions	+1	0	-1	-2	-3	-4	-5
5. When not paying attention	+1	0	-1	-2	-3	-4	-5
6. When involved with other activities, i.e., coloring, reading, etc	+1	0	-1	-2	-3	-4	-5.
7. When listening with a group of children	+1	0	-1	-2	-3	-4	-5

COMMENTS:

QUIET

TOTAL CONDITION SCORE [ ]

If listening in a quiet room (others may be present, but are being quiet), this child has difficulty hearing and understanding compared to other children of similar age and background.

8. When paying attention	+1	0	-1	-2	-3	-4	-5
9. When being asked a question	+1	0	-1	-2	-3	-4	-5
10. When being given simple instructions	+1	0	-1	-2	-3	-4	-5
11. When being given complicated, multiple instructions	+1	0	-1	-2	-3	-4	-5
12. When not paying attention	+1	0	-1	-2	-3	-4	-5
13. When involved with other activities, i.e., coloring reading, etc.	+1	0	-1	-2	-3	-4	-5
14. When listening with a group of children	+1	0	-1	-2	-3	-4	-5

COMMENTS:

IDEAL

TOTAL CONDITION SCORE [ ]

When listening in a quiet room, no distractions, face-to-face, and with good eye contact, this child has difficulty hearing an understanding compared to other children of similar age and background.

15. When being asked a question	+1	0	-1	-2	-3	-4	-5
16. When being given simple instructions	+1	0	-1	-2	-3	-4	-5
17. When being given complicated, multiple instructions	+1	0	-1	-2	-3	-4	-5

COMMENTS:

MULTIPLE INPUTS

TOTAL CONDITION SCORE [ ]

When, in addition to listening, there is also some other form of input, (i.e., visual, tactile, etc.) this child has difficulty hearing and understanding compared to other children of similar age and background.

18. When listening and watching the speaker's face	+1	0	-1	-2	-3	-4	-5
19. When listening and reading along when material is read aloud by another	+1	0	-1	-2	-3	-4	-5
20. When listening and watching someone provide an illustration, such as a model, drawing, information on the overhead projector or chalkboard, etc.	+1	0	-1	-2	-3	-4	-5

COMMENTS:

LISTENING CONDITION

		LESS DIFFICULTY	SAME AMOUNT	SLIGHTLY MORE	MORE DIFFICULTY	CONSID. MORE	SIGNIFIC. MORE	CAN'T FUNCTION
AUDITORY MEMORY SEQUENCING TOTAL CONDITION SCORE	If required to recall spoken information, this child has difficulty hearing and understanding compared to other children of similar age and background							
	21. Immediately recalling information such as a word, word spelling, numbers	+1	0	-1	-2	-3	-4	-5
	22. Immediately recalling simple instructions	+1	0	-1	-2	-3	-4	-5
	23. Immediately recalling multiple instructions	+1	0	-1	-2	-3	-4	-5
	24. Not only recalling information, but also the order and sequence of the information	+1	0	-1	-2	-3	-4	-5
	25. When delayed recollection (1 hour or more) of words, word spelling, numbers, etc. is required	+1	0	-1	-2	-3	-4	-5
	26. When delayed recollection (1 hour or more) of simple instructions is required	+1	0	-1	-2	-3	-4	-5.
	27. When delayed recollection (1 hour or more) of multiple instructions is required	+1	0	-1	-2	-3	-4	-5
	28. When delayed recollection (24 hours or more) is required	+1	0	-1	-2	-3	-4	-5
	COMMENTS:							
AUDITORY ATTENTION SPAN TOTAL CONDITION SCORE	If extended periods of listening are required, this child has difficulty paying attention, that is, being attentive to what is being said compared to other children of similar age and background.							
	29. When the listening time is less than 5 minutes	+1	0	-1	-2	-3	-4	-5
	30. When the listening time is 5-10 minutes	+1	0	-1	-2	-3	-4	-5
	31. When the listening time is over 10 minutes	+1	0	-1	-2	-3	-4	-5
	32. When listening in a quiet room	+1	0	-1	-2	-3	-4	-5
	33. When listening in a noisy room	+1	0	-1	-2	-3	-4	-5
	34. When listening first thing in the morning	+1	0	-1	-2	-3	-4	-5
	35. When listening near the end of the day, i.e., before supper time	+1	0	-1	-2	-3	-4	-5
	36. When listening in a room where there are also visual distractions	+1	0	-1	-2	-3	-4	-5
	COMMENTS:							

SCORING: The CHAPS can be scored two ways. Add the circled responses for each condition and place the sum in the Total Condition Score box in under each listed listening condition. Be careful to note "+" and "-" values when adding. Transcribe these sums as indicated below and determine the average score for each listening condition. The Total Condition Scores can be compared to the indicated PASS and FAIL ranges and the appropriate box checked. In addition, the average condition scores can be plotted on the graph to display performance as compared to the normal range. See the CHAPS manual for more complete validity and interpretation information.

LISTENING CONDITION	TOTAL CONDITION SCORE		AVERAGE CONDITION SCORE		
NOISE	_____	÷ 7 =	_____	Pass	Risk
QUIET	_____	÷ 7 =	_____	Pass	Risk
IDEAL	_____	÷ 3 =	_____	Pass	Risk
MULTIPLE	_____	÷ 3 =	_____	Pass	Risk
MEMORY	_____	÷ 8 =	_____	Pass	Risk
ATTENTION	_____	÷ 8 =	_____	Pass	Risk
TOTAL	_____	÷ 36 =	_____	Pass	Risk

TOTAL CONDITION SCORE:
PASS RANGE +36 to -11
AT-RISK RANGE -12 to -130

CHAPS Listening Condition Analysis: Transfer Average Condition Scores by entering "X" on graph (round 0.5 scores up to next decimal).

	NOISE	QUIET	IDEAL	MULT	MEM	ATTN	TOTAL
+1.0							
+0.5							
0.0			N O R M A L				
-0.5							
-1.0							
-1.5							
-2.0							
-2.5							
-3.0			A T - R I S K				
-3.5							
-4.0							
-4.5							
-5.0							

NOTE: Children who score in the at-risk range on the CHAPS will not necessarily require a special academic support program in school. Research found that 45% of students scoring in the at-risk range required no special support services. 50% of students scoring in the at-risk range had below grade level reading ability. 55% required some type of special support or accommodations to achieve success in school.

CLASSROOM ACOUSTICAL MODIFICATION EFFICACY SCALE I (CES-1)
Carl C. Crandell, Ph.D., Joseph J. Smaldino, Ph.D., and Brian M. Kreisman, Ph.D.

Teacher's Name: _____ **Date:** _____

Grade Level (Circle One): K   1   2   3   4   5   6   7   8   9   10   11   12

Class Size: _____ students

Classroom Setting (Check one): ☐ Regular   ☐ Special

Class Topic Area(s) (e.g., Reading, Math, History): _____

The acoustical modifications were recommended for (Check one):
   ☐ One Child   ☐ Several Children   ☐ Entire Classroom

The acoustical modifications were recommended for a child, or children, with the following auditory impairments (Check all that apply):
☐ hearing loss   ☐ developmental delay   ☐ English as a second language
☐ learning disability   ☐ attention disorder   ☐ auditory processing disorder
☐ speech/language delay ☐ dyslexia   ☐ young child (<15 years old)
☐ other _____

SECTION I:	**Please complete this section PRIOR to the acoustical modifications in the classroom.**

Instructions: Please list, in order of importance to you, four specific listening and/or learning needs that may exist in your classroom for which you would like to see improvement. Be as specific as possible and list at least four needs areas. (Example: I want the children to listen to me better when I am reading them a story.)

NEED AREA #1: _____
_____

NEED AREA #2: _____
_____

NEED AREA #3: _____
_____

NEED AREA #4: _____
_____

Do you have any concerns about acoustical modifications in your classroom?
(Check one): ☐ Yes   ☐ No

If yes, please note your concerns here:

Reprinted by permission of the authors.

212

Date:_____

The acoustical modifications have been present for _____ month(s).

What type of acoustical modifications were implemented (Check all that apply):
☐ acoustical ceiling tile installed
☐ acoustical wall tile installed
☐ carpeting installed
☐ draperies installed
☐ repaired/refurbished HVAC system
☐ repaired/refurbished lighting fixtures
☐ relocation of room
☐ relocation of children from noise source
☐ wall modification or repair
☐ ceiling modification or repair
☐ window modification or repair
☐ modifications of hallways
☐ acoustical furniture installed
☐ outside landscaping conducted
☐ other _____

Instructions: For each of the listening and/or learning needs that you identified in Section I, please indicate the degree of change (if any) observed in the need area on a scale from 1 to 7 (1 = the acoustical modifications made the need area much worse and 7 = the acoustical modifications made the need area much better).

	Much Worse	Worse	Slightly Worse	No Difference	Slightly Better	Better	Much Better
NEED AREA #1:	1	2	3	4	5	6	7
NEED AREA #2:	1	2	3	4	5	6	7
NEED AREA #3:	1	2	3	4	5	6	7
NEED AREA #4:	1	2	3	4	5	6	7

Do you still have any concerns about classroom modifications?
(Check one): ☐ Yes ☐ No

Please note any concerns or comments here:

FM AMPLIFICATION EFFICACY SCALE I   (FES-1)

Carl C. Crandell, Ph.D., Joseph J. Smaldino, Ph.D., and Brian M. Kreisman, Ph.D.

Teacher's Name: _____ **Date:** _____

Grade Level (Circle One):   K   1   2   3   4   5   6   7   8   9   10   11   12

Class Size: _____ students

Classroom Setting (Check one):   ☐ Regular   ☐ Special

Class Topic Area(s) (e.g., Reading, Math, History): _____

The FM system was recommended for (Check one):
☐ One Child   ☐ Several Children   ☐ Entire Classroom

The FM system was recommended for a child, or children, with the following:
(Check all that apply):
☐ hearing loss   ☐ developmental delay   ☐ English as a second language
☐ learning disability   ☐ attention disorder   ☐ auditory processing disorder
☐ speech/language delay   ☐ dyslexia   ☐ other _____

SECTION I:	Please complete this section PRIOR to using the personal FM system in the classroom.

Instructions: Please list, in order of importance to you, four specific listening and/or learning needs that may exist in your classroom for which you would like to see improvement. Be as specific as possible and list at least four needs areas. (Example: I want the child/children to listen to me better when I am reading them a story.)

NEED AREA #1: _____
_____

NEED AREA #2: _____
_____

NEED AREA #3: _____
_____

NEED AREA #4: _____
_____

Do you have any concerns about placing FM technology in your classroom?
(Check one):   ☐ Yes   ☐ No

If yes, please note your concerns here:

_____

Reprinted by permission of the authors.

Date:_____

The FM amplification system has been used for _____ month(s).

What type of microphone was used (Check one):
    ☐ Boom ☐ Lapel   ☐ Collar   ☐ Other _____

What type of FM system was used in the classroom (Check one)?

☐ Behind the ear FM   ☐ Personal FM with headphones
☐ Personal FM with silhouette   ☐ Personal FM with ear buds
☐ Personal FM and hearing aid (DAI)   ☐ "audio boot" coupled to hearing aid
☐ Personal FM and hearing aids   ☐ Tabletop/Desktop FM system
    (Induction loop/telecoil)
☐ Other _____

Instructions: For each of the listening and/or learning needs that you identified in Section I, please indicate the degree of change (if any) observed in the need area on a scale from 1 to 7 (1 = the FM system made the need area much worse and 7 = the FM system made the need area much better).

	Much Worse	Worse	Slightly Worse	No Difference	Slightly Better	Better	Much Better
NEED AREA #1:	1	2	3	4	5	6	7
NEED AREA #2:	1	2	3	4	5	6	7
NEED AREA #3:	1	2	3	4	5	6	7
NEED AREA #4:	1	2	3	4	5	6	7

Do you still have any concerns about FM technology?
(Check one): ☐ Yes   ☐ No

Please note any concerns or comments here:

SOUND FIELD AMPLIFICATION EFFICACY SCALE I (SES-1)

Carl C. Crandell, Ph.D., Joseph J. Smaldino, Ph.D., and Brian M. Kreisman, Ph.D.

Teacher's Name: _____ **Date:** _____

Grade Level (Circle One): K 1 2 3 4 5 6 7 8 9 10 11 12

Class Size: _____ students
Classroom Setting (Check one): ☐ Regular   ☐ Special
Class Topic Area(s) (e.g., Reading, Math, History): _____

The sound field FM system was recommended for (Check one):
    ☐ One Child   ☐ Several Children   ☐ Entire Classroom

The sound field FM system was recommended for a child, or children, with the following auditory impairments (Check all that apply):

☐ hearing loss   ☐ developmental delay   ☐ English as a second language
☐ learning disability   ☐ attention disorder   ☐ auditory processing disorder
☐ speech/language delay ☐ dyslexia   ☐ other _____

SECTION I: **Please complete this section PRIOR to the installation of the sound field FM system in the classroom.**

Instructions: Please list, in order of importance to you, four specific listening and/or learning needs that may exist in your classroom for which you would like to see improvement. Be as specific as possible and list at least four needs areas. (Example: I want the children to listen to me better when I am reading them a story.)

NEED AREA #1: _____
_____

NEED AREA #2: _____
_____

NEED AREA #3: _____
_____

NEED AREA #4 _____
_____

Do you have any concerns about placing sound field technology in your classroom?
(Check one): ☐ Yes   ☐ No   **If yes, please note your concerns below:**

216

SECTION II:	Please complete this section __AFTER__ using the sound field FM system at least one month.

Date:_____

The sound field FM amplification system has been used for _____ month(s)

What type of microphone was used (Check one):
  ☐ Boom ☐ Lapel ☐ Collar ☐ Other _____

How many loudspeakers were used in the classroom (Check one):
          ☐ One
          ☐ Two
          ☐ Three
          ☐ Four
          ☐ Ceiling Speaker used
          ☐ Desktop Unit used
          ☐ Other _____

Instructions: For each of the listening and/or learning needs that you identified in Section I, please indicate the degree of change (if any) observed in the need area on a scale from 1 to 7 (1 = the sound field system made the need area much worse and 7 = the sound field system made the need area much better).

	Much Worse	Worse	Slightly Worse	No Difference	Slightly Better	Better	Much Better
NEED AREA #1:	1	2	3	4	5	6	7
NEED AREA #2:	1	2	3	4	5	6	7
NEED AREA #3:	1	2	3	4	5	6	7
NEED AREA #4:	1	2	3	4	5	6	7

Do you still have any concerns about sound field technology?
(Check one): ☐ Yes   ☐ No

Please note any concerns or comments here:

CHAPTER 11

Marketing and Obtaining Funding for Sound Field Amplification

Laurie A. Allen, MA
Karen L. Anderson, PhD

KEY POINTS

- The very success and proliferation of sound field amplification use in the classroom can be perceived as a threat to budget-conscious school administrators and therefore should be marketed effectively in the schools.
- It is necessary to sit down with the building administrator and describe the use and benefits of sound field amplification equipment.
- Classroom size, shape, and acoustic treatment can vary from room to room; therefore, it is always prudent to have several teacher candidates to help facilitate matching the right equipment with the teachers and the needs of their classrooms.
- There are points to consider when selecting a teacher to try a sound field system in her or his classroom, such as select a teacher who appears to have a real desire to use the equipment, look for a teacher who is articulate and respected by his or her peers, and select a teacher who welcomes visitors to the classroom and who is willing to provide you with feedback.
- It is important to choose a classroom that has several factors undermining the listening environment, such as the teacher with the exceptionally soft voice, the room with many students, a large number of English as a second language (ESL) students, or a physically large or noisy classroom where amplification equipment will have the greatest impact.

- Once the parameters and personnel of the pilot project have been determined and any necessary parent permissions have been obtained, equipment installation and training can take place and data collection can begin.
- With classroom amplification providing a broad impact to student achievement and teacher health, numerous sources may be utilized for financial assistance, including grants from the school district.
- Once data has been collected to prove that the sound field classroom amplification is beneficial, share this information with local school board members, directors or coordinators of special education, the state superintendent of public instruction, local principals, and local service organizations.

The concept of sound field amplification has been promoted since the Mainstream Amplification Resource Room Study (MARRS) first became a U.S. Department of Education National Diffusion Network (NDN) project in 1979. The efforts of the NDN project were primarily aimed at educators as a way to improve educational effectiveness for students with undetected hearing impairment or other children with attention or auditory learning problems. The MARRS project revealed that all learners, including those who did not pass a 15 dB hearing screening, had increased levels of academic achievement compared to learners in unamplified classrooms. During the last decade, audiologists have become interested in using sound field amplification for students with recurrent otitis media, auditory processing disorders, or mild hearing loss in one or both ears. This interest has hastened the creation of classroom amplification systems in a variety of configurations and prices. Equipment is now more flexible and can be used in numerous settings in the educational arena.

As stated in previous chapters, the use of sound field classroom amplification is beneficial to students and teachers. Despite this finding, not every principal or superintendent welcomes equipment that teachers will fight to keep once they have used it. In other words, the very success and proliferation of sound field amplification use in the classroom can be perceived as a threat to budget-conscious school administrators. This chapter will thus examine how sound field amplification can be marketed effectively in the schools.

MARKETING PREPARATION

Preparation is the key to the successful introduction of sound field classroom amplification equipment. Initial legwork must be done to successfully promote the technology. Steps to follow (in this order) include:

1. A receptive school must be found with an administrator who is excited about the equipment.

2. Teachers must be selected to try the equipment for a pilot study.
3. The appropriate equipment must be selected to meet the physical needs of the classroom.
4. Appropriate teacher in-service training must be provided so that the staff is aware of the purpose of the equipment and how it is to be handled and used.
5. Data supporting the subjective and objective benefits of the use of sound field classroom amplification must be collected.

Once these steps are successfully completed, the concept of using amplification equipment typically sells itself.

GETTING STARTED: INITIATING A PILOT PROJECT

The following section discusses the needed steps of initiating a pilot project.

School Selection

In every school district, there are usually a few school principals who thrive on trying innovative programs or teaching methods in their buildings. In addition, there is often active parent participation and community support visible in these schools; they are the schools that are featured in local newspaper articles or photographs. This newspaper coverage is an indication that there is a school principal who likes to be educationally progressive and who wants the public to know about all of the interesting activities going on in the school building. This type of administrator represents a good candidate to approach regarding the use of sound field classroom amplification.

It is necessary to sit down with the building administrator and describe the use and benefits of sound field amplification equipment. Also helpful is providing a written summary of the sound field amplification concept and benefits. If possible, provide the principal with the name and telephone number of other administrators who have had experience with the equipment. After presenting the benefits of sound field amplification, ask the principal if he or she would be willing to try this type of equipment in one of the classrooms. If the principal seems receptive to the idea of trying the equipment, suggest that he or she conduct a small study of a single student or the performance and achievement of students in several classrooms to compare the effects in classrooms both with and without the amplification. Acknowledge that parent permission requirements will need to be respected and that test time-lines to gather data would need to be determined so that data collection could occur as conveniently as possible. Brainstorm which teachers the principal could identify as good candidates to approach to try the sound field amplification concept in the school.

Teacher Selection

Once a receptive school administrator has been identified, it is important to identify one or more teachers who are willing and excited to try the equipment. Classroom size, shape, and acoustic treatment can vary from room to room; therefore, it is always prudent to have several candidates to help facilitate matching the right equipment with the teachers and the needs of their classrooms. If possible, discuss the sound field amplification concept with the teachers whom the principal selected, preferably within their classrooms. In this way, you will be able to quickly form an idea about which rooms would benefit the most from the use of the equipment. Discuss the acoustic conditions in the classroom as you talk with the teachers about sound field amplification. Teachers are often very aware of annoying sound sources in the classroom that interfere with teaching activities. This firsthand information about the classrooms and the teachers' willingness to try the equipment will facilitate the selection process.

Consider the following points when selecting a teacher:

- Select a teacher who appears to have a real desire to use the equipment. Avoid forcing the use of the equipment on anyone. If the teacher tells you she has a strong voice that carries well, she is really trying to tell you that she is not interested. It will be better to find a different teacher to try the equipment rather than try to educate the defensive teacher about sound degradation across distance. She may eventually be open to the idea of trying the equipment, but it may be only after a colleague has used the sound field amplification equipment and reports back positively. If the principal suggests Teacher A and you find that this person is not receptive to the idea, go back to the principal and diplomatically suggest other possible candidates. Perhaps the room with high noise levels (e.g., buzzing lights) or a teacher with a soft voice would be a more logical choice. This way, the principal will learn that the equipment can be used in a variety of classrooms and will still have a say in the teacher-selection process.
- Look for the teacher who is articulate and respected by his or her peers. The sound field amplification equipment, if installed and maintained properly, will promote the benefits of improved classroom listening by itself. A well-respected, articulate teacher can do much to speed the promotion process at the school district and the community levels.
- Select a teacher who welcomes visitors to the classroom. Once you have the amplification system installed, you want people such as the school superintendent, PTA president, or a local newspaper reporter to come and experience the difference that the amplification can make in the classroom setting.
- Select a teacher who is willing to provide you with feedback. The teacher needs to know that you will be asking for his or her feedback

on the trial period. Feedback is typically acquired using questionnaires such as the teacher appraisal form of the Listening Inventory For Education (LIFE) (Anderson & Smaldino, 1998) or, if a specific student is targeted, the Screening Instrument for Targeting Educational Risk (SIFTER) (Anderson, 1989), or the Children's Auditory Performance Scale (CHAPS) (Smoski, Brunt, & Tannahill, 1998) can be completed and returned to you following the sound field amplification trial period (see Appendix 10-A).

Classroom Selection

Once you have a list of volunteer teachers, selection of an appropriate classroom needs to be carefully considered. Some questions to consider during the selection process include:

- The use of sound field classroom amplification will improve the signal-to-noise levels in classrooms, but it will not overcome the acoustical smearing effects of excessive reverberation. Therefore, it is important to consider if the reverberation time in the room is at an acceptable level to allow effective use of sound field classroom amplification. If the reverberation time is in excess of 0.6 second or if there is perceptible acoustic smearing of the speech signal, the room is not acceptable for sound field classroom amplification use.
- Can all of the speakers in the system be used in this room without having speaker wire draped across the travel paths in the room? Four speakers provide a direct sound signal to more students than just one or two speakers do.
- How many electrical outlets are available for use? Some systems require more than one outlet for the receiver or amplifier. Other brands require that each speaker be plugged into an outlet (and then no speaker wires are used). Be sure to consult with the teacher to find out which outlets in the classroom are available for use and where they are located.
- Are there places where speakers can be set or mounted so that they provide appropriate sound coverage throughout the room (e.g., one per wall rather than all speakers along one or two walls)?
- Is there a location where the receiver or amplifier can be placed so that it is away from excessive heat, cold, sinks, aquariums, and computers?
- Can one person (frequently the educational audiologist or hearing specialist in the school building) install the equipment, or will school district personnel be required to help (e.g., custodian, buildings and grounds electrician)?

Choosing a classroom where the amplification equipment will have the greatest impact is an important consideration. The amplification will be in use only for large group instruction; thus, avoid classrooms that have a small number of students who receive mostly one-to-one or small group instruction. Try to choose a room with several factors that undermine the listening environment, such as the teacher with the exceptionally soft voice, the room with many students, a large number of English as a second language (ESL) students, a physically large room, or a noisy classroom. Be sure to demonstrate to the teachers and any visitors the difference in the listening environment when the system is on and off.

Equipment Selection

Several companies manufacture sound field classroom amplification systems. These systems vary in features, price, and user-friendliness. The easiest way to obtain equipment for short-term use is to contact the manufacturers directly. All companies currently allow demonstration units to be placed in a school for at least a thirty-day trial period. Companies typically will require some type of written request or a purchase order on file. If a purchase order is required, it is important to realize that the district will not be billed for the equipment until the agreed-upon trial period has been completed. Sometimes trial periods can be scheduled sequentially so that different brands of equipment can be tried by the same teacher in order to allow comparison. Be aware that each individual system will require some additional teacher in-service training.

If you have limited experience with sound field amplification and it is not possible to carry out several trials of different equipment (i.e., exploring benefits of infrared versus FM types of equipment), then ask the manufacturers for names and telephone numbers of satisfied customers. Specifically request the names of people who do more than just sell the equipment to schools. Someone such as an educational audiologist or a teacher who has had the experience of installing and maintaining the equipment on a regular basis will provide valuable information. A testimony from a satisfied equipment user is very valuable when selecting which types of equipment to request for a demonstration trial period.

Manufacturers typically provide support people who are very helpful in assisting new users in the selection of appropriate devices. It may be possible to fax or email a digital picture or written sketch to assist in your discussion with the manufacturer.

Once the trial period is completed and a funding source for the equipment has been identified, select a single vendor for all systems in your district if possible. Not only will you establish a longtime relationship with the customer support people in just one company, you will also have to deal with providing spare parts for just one type of equipment. This will save you time and confusion.

When returning demonstration equipment to the manufacturer, take care to ensure that you use a reputable shipping service that provides a tracking number. This way, if there is a delay in the manufacturer receiving the returned equipment, you can document that the return was initiated and that your district is not responsible for the cost of this equipment.

Teacher In-Service

The teacher and classroom have been selected and the trial equipment has been ordered. Ask the principal to arrange an in-service meeting with the teachers so that you can give them a brief overview of the equipment and why it is going to be tried in their building. This will provide the teacher who will be using the sound field amplification equipment with informed peers who will be interested in her or his experiences. See Chapter 1 for a sample teacher in-service outline.

Data Collection

Once the parameters and personnel of the pilot project have been determined and any necessary parent permissions have been obtained, equipment installation and training can take place and data collection can begin. Be sure to allow ample time to train the teacher thoroughly on use of the equipment. Plan to visit the classroom on a regular basis to troubleshoot any problems and to provide encouragement. A visit or a contact a few days after equipment installation is highly recommended. If the teacher sounds unsure or has questions about use, be prompt in providing her with an answer; make sure to visit the classroom. At the end of the project, it is critical to have the involved school staff and students complete an evaluation form (see Appendix 10-A). This subjective feedback information from your local school district teachers and student population is very meaningful to your school superintendent, PTA members, and local service organizations, which may very well be your future sources of funding for equipment. This local information along with the current research literature makes for a very convincing case when you are presenting to others in your community.

PROMOTING THE BENEFITS AND COST-EFFECTIVENESS OF SOUND FIELD CLASSROOM AMPLIFICATION

Anything that helps children learn in a cost-effective and positive way should be of interest to all educators and parents; however, the bottom line will always be funding. Where will the school obtain the money to pay for the equipment? School administrators have difficulty when students and teachers are obviously benefiting from the equipment, it is wanted by all of the teachers, and the funds to purchase the equipment are not available.

Illustrating Cost Savings

One effective way to address cost savings is to provide administrators with projected cost savings for the district because of the use of the sound field amplification. Create a sample plan that includes a scenario for minimal and modest expansion. For example, if two classes each in kindergarten through second grade in a typical elementary school were amplified, it would cost approximately X amount of money as opposed to amplifying all kindergarten through second-grade classes, which would cost Y. Compare this expenditure to some other recognized cost, such as upgrading computers, installing carpeting, or projected substitute pay when a teacher takes days off because of maladies related to vocal abuse.

Use the growing body of available sound field amplification research (see Chapter 5) to develop cost-savings projections through decrease in special education needs (Educational Audiology Association, 1991). One excellent illustration of the impact of classroom amplification on special education comes from the Putnam County School District in Ohio (Phonic Ear, 1994). From 1985 to 1990, the district phased in sixty sound field amplification systems to help students with learning disabilities attend to verbal instruction more easily in the mainstreamed classroom setting. The cost of the amplification equipment at that time was approximately $1,500 per unit; however, some current brands are available at a lower cost. The number of students placed in learning disabilities (LD) programs declined nearly 40% (twenty-six students) during those five years. During 1990, the cost per year of placing a child in special education in Ohio was $2,600 (Berg, 1993). To continue the scenario into future years, we can predict that if Putnam County experiences another decline of twenty-six students placed in LD programs over another five-year period, the minimum savings at the end of the period would be as follows:

Cost of savings per year per potential LD student = $2,600.00
Number of school years not requiring special programming = 25
Total savings per student (keeping special education costs constant) = $13,000.00
Number of students not needing special education assistance because of amplification intervention (40% decline) = 226
Minimum savings over five-year time period = $338,000.00

Another means by which cost-effectiveness of sound field amplification equipment can be demonstrated is by comparing it to the expense per student of other classroom equipment. Rosenberg, Blake-Rahter, and Heavner (1995) compared the types of instructional delivery equipment in terms of the daily per person cost. The per-person cost was based on a class comprised of twenty-five students and one teacher and prorated for a five-year life of the equipment:

Instructional Equipment	Cost Per Pupil
FM Soundfield Classroom Amplification System	$0.14
FM Soundfield Classroom Amplification System with Boom Mic	$0.16
Computer with CD and Reference Bundle	$0.41
Basic Computer	$0.33
TV (25") with VCR	$0.18
Overhead Projector	$0.10
Filmstrip Projector with Sound	$0.08
Cassette Tape Player	$0.04

To be most effective, the technology specialist in your school or district could supply you with the prices of equipment that are in current use, including prices of equipment expansions (i.e., computer networks or upgrades). When you use this comparison, it is key to point out that the teacher typically uses sound field amplification during large group instruction throughout the school day, or approximately five hours per day. As instructional equipment, individual students rarely have more than a few minutes per day or week of instruction via the computer or television.

Funding Sound Field Amplification Equipment

Classroom amplification equipment is relatively inexpensive ($700–$1,000) and benefits both the students and the teachers. With classroom amplification providing a broad impact to student achievement and teacher health, numerous sources may be approached for financial assistance. If several amplification systems are desired, it would probably be best to write a grant to fund the equipment. Grant sources exist, but the competition between those applying for projects is often fierce and funding for the purchase of equipment is limited. In general, it is easier to find funding for an amount to support a small pilot project than for a large, district-wide project. Even a few thousand dollars is enough to fund a pilot project. If there is a person in charge of grant writing for your school district, contact her or him for advice. Grant sources can be found in reference books at your public and college libraries. It may be worthwhile to write a letter that contains one to two paragraphs describing your intended project (including time-line, district involvement, predicted outcome, and cost) and send the letter to many potential grant sources with a request for an application form if the project appears to be within their funding parameters. It may take a year to obtain funding, but if you inquire to a large number of potential sources, it is likely that several will be interested in your project and that funding will be received from at least one.

Once data is collected and analyzed, information about the benefits of sound field classroom amplification may be disseminated. First, share the information in a brief way with the local school board members and the director or coordinators of special education. Share your results with your state superintendent of public instruction. Be sure to send a copy to local principals.

Volunteer to talk to local service organizations; ask if they want to adopt a school or a classroom and provide the needed amplification equipment. Volunteer to write an article for the school newsletter or write a separate handout that the children can take home to their parents. Have stickers printed with "Amplification helps me hear better in school!" and pass them out to all of the students in the amplified rooms. Sport a large button on your lapel that says "Classroom amplification makes a difference." This will generate interest and questions. Push yourself to spread the word, because your efforts to promote the sound field amplification concept will result in positive gains for many children.

Another funding source can be the school's Parent Teacher Association (PTA). Equipment that has a direct positive impact on the children and the teachers has a very strong appeal to parent groups. Schools typically have fundraising activities throughout the year. Talking with the parent-teacher group, formalizing a plan of action, and advertising that some of the money will go to the purchase of amplification equipment provides a real incentive for parents to contribute. If you consider that the average cost of an amplification system is about $800, you can equate that to profits from two book fairs or four school bake sales for a school of four hundred to five hundred students. Perhaps a percentage of the profits from the lounge concession machines or from the school supply store could be earmarked for buying the amplification equipment. Finding a funding source is an opportunity for creativity!

If the school you wish to amplify does not have an active PTA, consider speaking to local service organizations (e.g., Sertoma, Lions Club, Rotary Club, etc.) or determine if the school has a business or corporate sponsor that would like to "adopt" a classroom or grade. Corporate sponsors may be willing to support a relatively low-cost, short-term, highly visible project. Even if only one system was purchased each year, there would be an amplified classroom at each grade level in seven years at a typical elementary school. Any assistance should be reported to the local newspaper, and perhaps a small plaque could be mounted on the equipment or outside the classroom stating the name of the organization or sponsor that provided the amplification equipment for the classroom.

Calling your local Chamber of Commerce or information and referral office may identify names of contact people for the service organizations.

THE SINGLE-STUDENT APPROACH

As an alternative to the pilot project approach for promotion, it is sometimes feasible to introduce sound field amplification into a school building by obtaining it for a student with recognized hearing needs. One could approach the use of the equipment for one student as an opportunity for the whole school staff to learn more about hearing loss and how sound field amplification can benefit students and teachers. Be aware, however, that if the equipment does not markedly benefit the student in question, it will be removed from the classroom even if the teacher loves it and the benefit is evident to the rest of the students. Inviting representatives from the parent-teacher organization to observe in the classroom and then to consider funding single units for use in the classrooms may be fruitful.

For the single-student approach, a likely candidate must be chosen. Choose student candidates carefully. Too many recommendations to any one principal or administration may cause your opinion to no longer be considered credible. Even in well-funded school districts, there are only so many dollars budgeted for anticipated equipment needs for students with special needs. With careful introduction to the use and benefits of this equipment, you can develop a vocal group of amplification supporters (teachers, principals, parents), and the budget for amplification equipment may increase slowly from year to year.

Our purpose in providing classroom amplification is to improve the students' listening environment so that they can learn as normally as possible. If the student is already perceived as a normal learner, it is difficult to be successful in promoting the amplification equipment to help him or her hear and, subsequently, learn better. Children who use hearing aids or cochlear implants require hearing technology that delivers the amplified speech at or relatively near ear-level; therefore, classroom sound field amplification is not the technology of choice for these students. Children with recognized attention and listening difficulties, histories of middle ear effusion, unilateral hearing loss, or auditory processing disorders can be considered candidates for the single-student approach. The functional abilities of the single-student approach candidate, such as student attention and class participation, should be discussed as areas of need as well as potential improvement in academic performance. To illustrate the level of difficulty a child is experiencing, obtain information from the classroom teacher about the child's performance prior to the use of classroom amplification. This information can be obtained by asking the teacher to complete a checklist such as the SIFTER, CHAPS, or Teacher Appraisal of the LIFE (see Appendix 10-A). In addition, the educational audiologist or educational hearing specialist could obtain information by performing a Functional Listening Evaluation (FLE) (Johnson & VonAlmen, 1997) of the child in the classroom or in a noisy environment similar to the classroom.

By working with the teacher to discuss the results of the SIFTER, CHAPS, LIFE, or FLE and describing sound field amplification equipment, it is possible to discover if the teacher would be willing, or preferably excited, to try sound field amplification for the benefit of the student and the class. If the teacher is not a willing participant during the trial period, the chances of the trial being successful and creating excitement about the sound amplification concept throughout the school is doubtful. Also, if the principal is not a strong supporter of the trial period and is not interested in the results of sound field amplification for all students, your efforts probably will not be successful. As with the pilot project approach, preparation is the key to success.

Case Study: Obtaining Funding for Sound Field Technology for General Education Classrooms

An elementary school in a large city district had been putting sound systems in a few of its classrooms based on the treatment model. That is, a child was identified with a hearing problem such as fluctuating hearing loss caused by otitis media with accompanying academic deficit, and a sound system subsequently was recommended and installed. Funding was obtained using special education monies.

Teachers in the amplified rooms started noticing that other children in the class also benefited from the sound field system. For example, children in one third-grade class demonstrated improvement in spelling scores. Children in an amplified second-grade classroom exhibited greater fluency when reading aloud using the pass-around microphone.

The principal, supported by the district's educational audiologist and the school's speech-language pathologist, decided to put sound field systems in every classroom. The problem was funding. Who would pay for sound systems in every room? The director of special education said that she had no funds for general education projects. Because the driving force behind the principal's decision was literacy and academic improvement rather than management of hearing loss, local foundations that supported literacy initiatives were petitioned.

One private city foundation liked the proposal and funded sound systems for all kindergarten and first-grade classrooms in the school. Following installation, local media were called and a story ran in area newspapers and on local TV stations.

Six months later, the audiologist contacted two prominent local businesses and successfully obtained funding for the third-grade classrooms. Once again, media were called and the story was reported. Plaques recognizing the granting foundation and the local businesses were hung in the entrance hallway.

This case study illustrates the point that there are multiple sources for funding when we use a universal designimperative (see Chapter 12) and link sound systems to literacy and to the No Child Left Behind Act of 2001 rather than to hearing loss. Also, there is great value in media and public recognition of funding sources such as foundations and local businesses.

SUMMARY

Sound field amplification has been in use in classrooms for at least twenty-five years. The concept of amplifying the teacher's voice so that all children can perceive verbal instruction without undue listening effort is good for teachers and good for children's achievement and behavior. With patience, information, and a willingness to assist schools in trying the equipment, we can achieve the worthy goal of sound field amplification in every classroom! A hearing loss simulation procedure that the authors have found helpful is included in Appendix 11-A.

DISCUSSION TOPICS

1. What are four points to consider when selecting a teacher to use a sound field system in her or his classroom?
2. What are factors that often make the classroom listening environment difficult for students? How can sound field amplification improve the listening environment?
3. Discuss three questions that should be addressed during the selection process of the classroom that will be using a sound field amplification system.
4. List four different sources that a school could approach for funding of a classroom amplification system.
5. Explain the single-student approach to amplification and describe the type of student who would not be a likely candidate for this approach.

REFERENCES

Anderson, K. (1989). *Screening Instrument for Targeting Education Risk (SIFTER)*. Tampa, FL: Educational Audiology Association.

Anderson, K., & Smaldino, J. (1998). *Listening Inventory for Education (LIFE)*. Tampa, FL: Educational Audiology Association.

Berg, F. (1993). *Acoustics and sound systems in schools*. Clifton Park, NY: Thomson Delmar Learning.

Educational Audiology Association. (1991). *Sound field classroom amplification: A collection of writings by members of the Educational Audiology Association*. Tampa, FL: Educational Audiology Association.

Johnson, C. D., & VonAlmen, P. (1997). The functional listening evaluation. In C. D. Johnson, P. V. Benson, & J. B. Seaton, (Eds.), *Educational audiology handbook*, Clifton Park, NY: Thomson Delmar Learning.

Northern, J., & Downs, M. (1991). *Hearing in children* (4th ed.). Baltimore: Williams & Wilkins.

Phonic Ear (1994). *Facts, figures & FM*. Petaluma, CA: Phonic Ear.

Rosenberg, G. G., Blake-Rahter, P., & Heavner, J. (1995, December). Enhancing listening and learning environments with FM soundfield classroom amplification. American Speech-Language-Hearing Association Annual Convention, Orlando, FL.

Smoski, W. J., Brunt, M. A., & Tannahill, J. C. (1998). *Children's Auditory Performance Scale (CHAPS)*. Tampa, FL: Educational Audiology Association.

APPENDIX 11-A
HEARING LOSS SIMULATION EXERCISE

A minimal hearing loss can be effectively simulated by asking participants to plug their ears with their fingers. Northern and Downs (1991) reported that by plugging your ears with your fingers, the following degrees of hearing loss would be imposed:

250 Hz	500 Hz	1,000 Hz	2,000 Hz	4,000 Hz	8,000 Hz
25 dB	25 dB	20 dB	20 dB	15 dB	15 dB

This degree of hearing loss approximates a typical hearing loss that accompanies middle ear effusion, which is common in young children. Hearing screening procedures performed in most schools would not always identify this degree of hearing loss. Finally, even the most optimally fit hearing aids rarely improve a child's hearing levels to this degree of loss. Even this minimal degree of hearing loss will interfere with the clarity of speech and the perception of high-pitch speech sounds that are critical for word recognition.

Exercise: Instruct participants that you will be reading a brief passage and that you want them to listen carefully, as there will be questions asked. Have all participants plug their ears with their fingers and keep them in that position until you notify them. Read the passage "Childhood Memories" using a typical teacher loudness. Vary your position in the room by standing and facing the group with your mouth clearly visible, turning to face the chalkboard, and roaming among the participants to all parts of the room. If you are demonstrating the effects of sound field amplification, start the simulation with the amplification off; turn it on for the middle portion, as indicated; and then turn it off again for the last third of the passage. Once you have finished reading the passage, instruct the participants to unplug their ears. If you have sound field amplification, turn it on again for the question portion. Proceed to ask the questions provided in the passage "Childhood Memories." Call on people with hands raised and also select people at random from all sections of the room. If the person you called on does not know the answer to your question, remind the person that he or she should have been paying attention while the short story was read.

Once the simulation and questions have been completed, start a discussion with the participants using the following questions:

1. How did you feel while you had the hearing loss?
2. What did you do when you couldn't understand what was being said?
3. What behaviors (e.g., daydreaming, frustration, tuning out, distraction by noises) do you think children with mild hearing loss exhibit in the classroom?

4. What accommodations (e.g., preferential seating, repeating important information from class discussions, checking for comprehension of new vocabulary and information, choosing a student buddy to help with directions and following classroom activities, limiting noise, facing students during instruction, etc.) should be made for these students in the classroom?

By experiencing this degree of hearing loss and generating their own list of behaviors and accommodations, participants are much more likely to remember and act on this information.

CHILDHOOD MEMORIES

A Story for Demonstrating the Effects of Minimal to Mild or Fluctuating Hearing Loss

By Laurie Allen, MA

When I was a little girl, my family would spend a week at a fishing resort in Minnesota. While my mother would pack our clothes, bed linens, and kitchen utensils, my father would work getting our little boat, the *Ripple,* ready for the lake. In the garage, he would make a big pile of all of the things we would need for our fishing trip. He had fishing poles, tackle boxes, life vests, seat cushions, a minnow bucket, a small outboard motor, a gas can, a container of earthworms, and a fishing net. He packed all of these things into our boat, which we pulled behind our big Ford car named Gertrude. Mother packed all of her things in Gertie's big trunk along with a roast chicken lunch for us to eat at the little park in St. Cloud, Minnesota.

(Turn sound field amplification on.)
We would try to have most everything packed the night before so that we could leave early in the morning. My mother would try to sneak some medicine into my morning juice so I would not get carsick, but I could always taste it. I told her that I couldn't taste it if she put it in chocolate milk. When we were ready to go, my father let my sister and I climb into the boat and ride to the end of our street. Although it was a very short ride, it was so much fun. At the end of the ride, we would climb out of the boat and get into the backseat of Gertie. My mother would draw an imaginary line with her finger across the midpoint of the backseat. She would say to us, "You stay on your half and you stay on your half." I was always envious of my sister because she could read in the car and not get sick. She would read most of the way, and I would get bored looking out of the window.

(Turn sound field amplification off.)

Sometimes along the way, we would sing to pass the time. My family would sing "Daisy, Daisy, Give me your answer do" or "You are my sunshine, my only sunshine." My mother would sing the harmony part, and we sounded so good. Other times we would play the alphabet game by searching for letters on billboards and signs. My sister and I liked to count Volkswagen cars and call them "peewee punches." Whenever you saw a peewee, you have to punch the other person. That was our favorite game, but my mother did not like it. She would turn around and draw that imaginary line again down the backseat.

1. Name at least four items that Father packed for the fishing trip. (unamplified)
2. What was the name of the little boat? (unamplified)
3. Where did Father pack his fishing supplies for the trip? (unamplified)
4. What did one sister do in the car that the other could not? (amplified)
5. What did the family do to pass the time while traveling? (unamplified)
6. Who was Gertie? (unamplified)
7. What kind of car is a peewee car? (unamplified)
8. Why did Mother draw an imaginary line on the backseat? (amplified)
9. What did the girls get to do when the family started their vacation? (amplified)
10. The medicine was mixed into what beverage? (amplified)

_____

CHAPTER 12

Laws and Regulations That Govern the Utilization of Sound Field Amplification

Carol Flexer, PhD

KEY POINTS

- Universal design, a concept consistent with legislative mandates, means that the assistive technology is not specially designed for an individual student but rather for a wide range of students. Universally designed approaches are implemented by general education teachers rather than by special education teachers.
- Special education is a failure-based system; a child needs to be failing and keep failing in order to qualify for special education services.
- Four main federal laws mandate audiologic services for infants and children, and all four federal laws require that children with disabilities have equal access to a free appropriate public education (FAPE).
- The Technology-Related Assistance Act for Individuals with Disabilities Amendments of 1994 provides access to assistive technology services and devices for individuals with disabilities of all ages; therefore, this act could be a source of funds for sound field technology for students with disabilities in both special education and general education classrooms.
- The No Child Left Behind Act of 2001 (NCLB) requires schools to show adequate yearly progress (AYP) toward meeting the goal of 100% proficiency in reading and math for all students in third through eighth grades by 2012; by improving the signal-to-noise ratio and enhancing acoustic accessibility, sound field technology can provide the evidence-based outcomes needed for school districts to be in compliance with NCLB.
- When recommending sound field systems from a treatment paradigm perspective, the need for the technology must be documented by an objective measure.

As mentioned in Chapter 1, amplification technologies such as hearing aids, personal FM systems, and now cochlear implants historically have been recommended as treatments for hearing loss; thus, their use in school fell under the purview of special education legislation. Because there certainly are populations for whom an enhanced signal-to-noise ratio can mean the difference between passing and failing in school, sound field technologies typically have been included in the treatment or special education category for hearing problems. If viewed as a treatment, sound field technology is recommended on a case-by-case basis.

At this point, it is critical to emphasize that sound field systems are not replacements for personal-worn FM systems. Many children who wear hearing aids continue to need the superior signal-to-noise ratio provided by personal-worn FM systems that channel the signal directly from the talker through the hearing aids to the brain of the listener.

Both sound field distribution systems and personal FM systems can be used effectively in the same room. In many instances, using both at the same time can create the best listening and learning environment because each serves a different purpose. The sound field distribution system, appropriately installed and used in a mainstream classroom, improves and equalizes acoustic access for all pupils and creates a "listening" in the room. The individual-worn FM system allows the particular child with hearing aids to have the most favorable signal-to-noise ratio. The teacher need wear only a single microphone or transmitter if the sound field unit and the individual FM are on the same radio frequency, or if the personal-worn FM transmitter can be coupled to the sound field amplifier.

UNDERSTANDING SOUND FIELD TECHNOLOGY FROM A UNIVERSAL DESIGN RATHER THAN FROM A TREATMENT PERSPECTIVE

With the recognition that all children require an enhanced signal-to-noise ratio comes the necessity of moving beyond recommending sound field technology on a case-by-case basis as a treatment for hearing problems. Rather, sound field distribution systems need to be integrated into the general education arena. The concept of universal design can be useful in this regard.

The idea of universal design originated in the architectural domain with the common examples of curb cuts, ramps, and automatic doors. After years of use, it was found that the modifications that were originally believed to be relevant for only a few people turned out to be useful and beneficial for a large percentage of the population.

The concept of universal design has been defined as the design of products and environments so that they are useable by all people, to the greatest extent possible, without the need for adaptation or specialized design (Bremer, Clapper, Hitchcock, Hall, & Kachgal, 2002). In other words, universal design is preemptive. If an environment is designed correctly to begin with, additional accommodations will be unnecessary.

A major reason for the emphasis on designs that benefit everyone is to avoid stigmatizing or segregating people who need the universal design feature (Wehmeyer, Lance, & Bashinski, 2002). If students feel singled out or stigmatized, they may not be motivated to use the equipment, independent of whether or not the equipment is effective (Bowe, 2000).

In terms of learning, universal design means that the assistive technology is not specially designed for an individual student but rather for a wide range of students. Universally designed approaches are implemented by general education teachers rather than by special education teachers ("Universal design," 1999).

OVERVIEW OF FEDERAL LAWS

Even though universal design is the most sensible way to allow acoustic accessibility for all children from the outset, there are bound to be some children who must have a very favorable signal-to-noise ratio and who will not automatically be in classes that contain sound distribution systems. Such children will benefit from special education legislation and accessibility legislation.

Special education is a failure-based system. A child qualifies for special education services when it has been documented that the child is unable to benefit from the standard classroom and typical curricular process (Flexer, 1999). That is, a child needs to be failing in the general education system in order to be eligible to receive special education services (Seaver, 2003). Moreover, the child must keep failing in order for special education services to be maintained. Special education is not a prevention-based system. It is a failure-based system.

Four main federal laws have evolved over the last thirty-one years that mandate audiologic services for infants and children: The Education for All Handicapped Children Act of 1975 (the original Public Law 94-142); an updated version of 94-142 called the Education of the Handicapped Act Amendments of 1986 (Public Law 99-457); the most recent version called the Individuals with Disabilities Education Act (IDEA) Amendments of 1997 (Public Law 105-17); and the Rehabilitation Act of 1973 (specifically, Section 504), a civil rights act that focuses on accessibility. All four federal laws require that children with disabilities have equal access to a free appropriate public education (FAPE) (Ackerhalt & Wright, 2003). In addition, the Technology-Related Assistance Act of 1994 and the No Child Left Behind Act of 2001 have potential connection to the use of sound field and the concept of universal design.

Public Law 94-142 (Special Education)

Public Law 94-142 (now called IDEA) also is known as the Education for All Handicapped Children Act of 1975. This law is the cornerstone of special education and provides four basic rights for children with disabilities. PL 94-142 mandates the following:

- Each child with a suspected disability is entitled to a thorough assessment of the nature and degree of a specific disability.
- Children with disabilities are entitled to a free and appropriate public education from the ages of three years through twenty-one years.
- This education is to be provided by placement in the least restrictive environment (LRE), giving maximum emphasis to, whenever possible, placing the child with disabilities among children who are not disabled, a process known as mainstreaming.
- These children are entitled to supplementary aids and services (related services) to ensure that their educational program as stipulated in an Individualized Educational Program (IEP) will be successful. The IEP is a legal written contract, developed by the school and parents, that specifies instructional and related services needed for the child to obtain an appropriate education.

Related services are developmental, corrective, and other supportive services required to assist a child who is disabled to benefit from special education and include:

- transportation
- audiological services
- speech/language therapy
- psychological services
- physical and occupational therapy
- recreation (including therapeutic recreation), social work services, medical services (for diagnostic and evaluation purposes only), and counseling services
- early identification and assessment of disabilities
- school health services
- parent counseling and training

PL 94-142 further protects the rights of parents and guarantees due process in classification and program placement for the child. Due process is a legal procedure designed to settle disagreements among parents, guardians, and the school district when problems arise about any aspect of special education or related services. A due process proceeding generally is initiated by the parents of a child with a disability when less formal solutions, such as mediation, have not worked.

One component of this extensive law pertains to audiology. As clarified in the Code of Federal Regulations on Education, Title 34, Section 300.13 (1986), audiology includes:

- Identification of children with hearing loss;
- Determination of the range (what frequencies or pitches are involved), nature (sensorineural, conduction, or mixed loss), and degree (mild, moderate, severe, profound) of hearing loss, including referral for medical or other professional (such as audiologists or speech pathologists) attention for the habilitation (helping the child form the basic capability to maximally use) of hearing;
- Provision of habilitative activities, such as language habilitation, auditory training, speech-reading (lipreading), hearing evaluation, and speech conversation;
- Creation and administration of programs for prevention of hearing loss;
- Counseling and guidance of pupils, parents, and teachers regarding hearing loss; and
- Determination of the child's need for group and individual amplification, selecting and fitting an appropriate hearing aid, and evaluating the effectiveness of amplification. (p. 14)

The Code of Federal Regulations on Education provides two definitions that continue to apply to children who are hearing impaired. These may be found in Title 34, Section 300.5, of the code (1986). The code defines deafness as a "hearing impairment which is so severe that the child is impaired in processing linguistic information through hearing with or without amplification, which adversely affects educational performance." The code further defines hard of hearing as a "hearing impairment, whether permanent or fluctuating, such as that experienced by children with ear infections, which adversely affects a child's educational performance but which is not included under the definition of deaf in this section" (p. 12).

The critical item to note in these definitions is that children with all degrees of hearing impairment, permanent or fluctuating, are entitled to audiologic rehabilitative services to support their educational performance—provided that their educational performance has been negatively affected by that hearing loss. Special education is a failure-based system, so failure must be documented.

Technology-Related Assistance Act of 1994

The Technology-Related Assistance Act for Individuals with Disabilities Amendments of 1994 provides access to assistive technology services and devices for individuals with disabilities of all ages. Devices are actual items or equipment, while a service is any effort that directly assists the child in selection, acquisition, or use of assistive technology devices. Assistive technology and services offer great promise for increasing, maintaining, and improving functioning in natural environments that are part of students' educational goals. While sound field technology is not specifically mentioned, it could be argued that sound field systems placed in general education classrooms could improve the function of students in that environment.

The act is a state-grants program, like much disability legislation. Grants are provided to develop a consumer responsive, comprehensive, state-wide program of technology-related assistance for individuals of all ages. A major part of the funding was used to finance the purchase of assistive technology devices and services. Therefore, this act could be a source of funds for sound field technology for students with disabilities in both special education and general education classrooms.

No Child Left Behind Act of 2001

The No Child Left Behind Act of 2001 (NCLB) was signed into law on January 8, 2002. This bill, which is a reauthorization of the Elementary and Secondary Education Act (ESEA), is perhaps the most significant federal education reform measure of the past three decades (Ruppmann, 2003). This act received unprecedented bipartisan support in regard to holding schools more accountable for the academic achievement of their students. In addition, this law attempts to address the achievement gap between wealthy majority and poor minority pupils. The provisions require schools to make genuine progress in closing the persistent achievement gaps between students who are disadvantaged or disabled and their peers. States now must account for the achievement of all public elementary and secondary school students in a manner that results in continuous and substantial improvement (Browder & Spooner, 2003).

NCLB focuses on the four major themes of school choice, standards, accountability, and testing. The federal government is working with the states to support and build on local and state efforts to improve education and guarantee yearly progress. Ultimately, the act sets national standards and requires student assessments by school districts to gauge districts' progress toward improving academic achievement. All children, including those with disabilities, will be impacted by these requirements (Browder & Spooner, 2003). Compliance with this law will require statutory changes by some states in order to bring state assessment and accountability systems into alignment with the new federal mandates.

State education agencies (SEAs) are to use Title I administrative funds to develop challenging academic content standards and academic assessments. In addition, SEAs must design policies to allow students who are at persistently dangerous pubic schools to attend safe public schools within the district. Private school students can continue to receive services from NCLB programs. Home schools are not subject to NCLB or to NCLB assessments.

Accountability through testing and high standards is the foundation of this authentic educational reform. NCLB mandates the tracking of each district's annual yearly progress (AYP). AYP is intended to ensure that every child learns, every school has the opportunity to improve, and every dollar is spent wisely for those purposes (Turnbull, Turnbull, Wehmeyer, & Park, 2003). NCLB requires the annual testing of children in third through eighth grades, at a minimum, in reading and math. States are allowed to design and select their own tests. The law gives states until the 2005–2006 school year to develop and implement math and reading tests for every child in third through eighth grades, and science must be assessed by the 2007–2008 school year (Ruppmann, 2003).

As discussed, NCLB requires schools to show AYP toward meeting the goal of 100% proficiency in reading and math for all students in third through eighth grades by 2012. Progress must be demonstrated each year. For example, a state cannot propose to make minimal improvement in student performance in the early years in anticipation of later dramatic gains in performance by the end of the twelve-year time-line (Browder & Spooner, 2003). Linear incremental improvement in student performance toward meeting the 100% proficiency for all students in the state by 2012 must be documented. It is important to note that NCLB regulations limit the use of alternate achievement standards to no more than 1% of all students in the grades that are assessed (Turnbull et al., 2003). Therefore, these accountability measures will likely create an even greater impetus than does IDEA of 1997 to link special education IEP goals with the content standards of the general education curriculum (President's Commission, 2002).

Even though NCLB primarily focuses on assessment and outcomes, a strong argument can be made that such measures cannot be achieved independent of the location and quality of instruction. For students with disabilities or for students who are disadvantaged, access to and inclusion in the culture and instruction of the general education classroom is an essential prerequisite to achieving the academic outcomes prescribed by the NCLB (LeRoy & Kulik, 2003). It therefore seems logical that equipping general education classrooms with sound field amplification from the outset, using a universal design imperative, can allow acoustic accessibility for diverse populations of learners.

To summarize, sound field amplification seems to mesh perfectly with NCLB. As noted in Chapter 5, there is ample evidence that sound field technology, appropriately installed and used, enhances pupils' performance and literacy development. School districts are desperate to find means of improving AYP for their students (Ruppmann, 2003). By improving the signal-to-noise ratio and enhancing acoustic accessibility, sound field technology can provide the evidence-based outcomes needed for school districts to be in compliance with NCLB.

IDEA of 1997 (Special Education)

Assuring that children with disabilities have the opportunity to be educated has evolved through laws that mandate certain educational rights. In addition, these laws have been amended twice since enactment in 1986 to address certain specific concerns that have arisen since the initial passage of Public Law 94-142. New amendments of this law are anticipated. Each reiteration of the disability law expands and strengthens previous legislation.

One change from earlier legislation that was included in IDEA of 1997 was that of greater attention to the general educational curriculum framework. This included assessment processes and planning as well as instructional activities. Special education now needs to make large efforts in ensuring participation of children with disabilities in state-wide performance tests and accountability systems. Within the IEP, annual instructional goals need to be referenced to the general education curriculum. General education teachers now need to participate in the IEP process. Improvement in results from adaptations and supports in the general education curriculum will take precedence over the past practices focusing on disability categories and remediation models.

With IDEA of 1997, related services were also available to help students participate in and benefit from education and activities in the classroom and community settings. Impairments or lack of technology to enhance learning environments may *not* be used as a reason for excluding students from the classes and curricula of their choice. Disability rights have to do with contributing to, participating in, and benefiting from activities in all aspects of community living, citizenship, and the pursuit of personal and career goals. Education is a basic right under the U.S. Constitution because without education one can neither fully exercise other rights nor realize the benefits of citizenship.

Because of the focus on the general education system, universal design comfortably fits into IDEA. The intent of IDEA's access to the general curriculum mandates was to ensure that all students with disabilities have access to and benefit from a challenging curriculum and are held to high standards and expectations (Bremer et al., 2002).

Section 504 of the Rehabilitation Act of 1973
(Typically Financed via General Education, Not Special Education, Funds)

Unlike special education legislation, this law is not based on failure; rather, it is predicated on accessibility. The law is a civil rights act that prohibits recipients (such as agencies and organizations) of federal funds from discriminating against "qualified individuals with disabilities in the United States." Specifically, a recipient of federal funds that operates a public elementary or secondary education program shall provide FAPE to each qualified person with a disability who is in the recipient's jurisdiction, regardless of the nature or severity of the person's disability. The emphasis in Section 504 is equal opportunity or equal access. Section 504 does not link the child's disability to his or her need for special education services but rather to the existence of limitations on a major life activity. On the other hand, IDEA requires that a child's disability be linked directly to the need for special education services in order to benefit from the educational process.

The Section 504 plan can outline access support with accommodations. However, its regulations are not as clearly defined or as financially supported as IDEA's. Any student who qualifies for an IEP automatically qualifies for a Section 504 plan, but the reverse is not true. In order to qualify, some documentation must be provided showing that equal access cannot be obtained without it.

SHOW THE NEED FOR TECHNOLOGY

The key to securing technology from the school system is to obtain data documenting need (Ackerhalt & Wright, 2003). A multifactored evaluation (MFE), which is a thorough evaluation by a multidisciplinary team, is necessary to document the need for a child to receive special services. The last category on most MFE forms is "Assistive Technology Needs." In order for assistive technology to be recommended within any legislative framework, some type of evaluation must be conducted. That is, can we document that the child in question cannot obtain an appropriate education unless sound field amplification is utilized? Can the child's failure in the regular education system be linked to hearing difficulties in the classroom? What tests can be administered to document listening difficulties in the classroom?

Perform Speech-in-Noise Sound Field Testing: One Way to Document Need

By adding only two speech tests to the basic audiometric test battery, an audiologist in a school or clinical setting can provide evidence that a child has a hearing problem that interferes with acoustic accessibility of classroom instruction. If a child's hearing problem limits acoustic accessibility, then by evoking Section 504 of the Rehabilitation Act of 1973 we can advocate in a proactive fashion for an appropriate classroom amplification system. That is, we do not have to wait until a child fails and is eligible for special education funding under IDEA of 1997 before we can provide services.

To provide functional information about acoustic accessibility, word-identification testing should be performed in the sound field in the unaided condition first (if the child wears hearing aids). If the child wears hearing aids, these same tests also can be performed in an aided condition. Appropriate speech stimuli for the language level of the child should be presented at the average loudness level that a child in a favorable classroom environment—45 dB HL—receives speech. Because the child also must hear soft speech, another list of words should be presented at 35 dB HL. If phonetically balanced (PB) words are presented only at 40 dB sensation level (SL) under earphones, functional information is not provided about accessibility to typical classroom instruction. Words presented at a loud level in perfect quiet always overestimate a child's auditory discrimination ability.

In addition, word identification testing in the sound field ought to be conducted at 45 dB HL using a +5 S/N ratio—a favorable noise level in a primary-level classroom (Berg, 1993). A child might appear to hear very well in the acoustically perfect environment of a sound room but have a great deal of trouble hearing in a typical classroom.

SCAN-C: A Normed Test That Can Be Administered to Document Need

The SCAN-C (Keith, 2000) was developed as a screening test for auditory processing disorders. However, there are two subtests, competing words and competing sentences, that can be used to provide some documentation of a child's classroom listening difficulty. These tests are normed on children from ages three through eleven. Remember, some documentation is necessary in order for any assistive device to be recommended.

Case Study Utilizing Federal Laws

A first-grade student with a long history of chronic and fluctuating hearing loss was referred to a community-based audiologist for an audiologic assessment. There was no educational audiologist in her school district, and her classroom did not have a sound distribution system. Academically, she was performing within the average range. She did not qualify for a multifactored evaluation because special education is a failure-based system, and this child was not yet failing. She did, however, appear frustrated in school by crying easily, having "illnesses" that kept her from school, and saying "what" a great deal.

Audiologic testing showed air conduction responses of 15–25 dB across thresholds (pure-tone average of 20 dB HL—"minimal" hearing loss), bone conduction thresholds were 0–10 dB HL, and tympanometry revealed negative middle ear pressure on the day of the test. Her history suggests that on some days she hears better, and on many days she hears worse. Word-identification testing, performed at the diagnostic level 40 dB SL (60 dB HL), revealed a score of 92% using a standardized word list. Note that 60 dB HL is a louder level than speech is typically heard in any classroom. Moreover, an audiologic sound suite is an acoustically perfect environment—vastly different from any classroom. Therefore, when functional testing was performed, she did much poorer. At 45 dB HL (average conversational level), her score declined to 78%, and when noise was added, her score further declined to 64%. At 35 dB HL, a soft level that is often the level of speech in a classroom, her score was 72%. Her scores on the competing words and competing sentences subtests of the SCAN-C were below the norm, continuing to document significant difficulty hearing in noise. The community-based audiologist requested that the teacher fill out the Fisher's Auditory Problems Checklist (Fisher, 1985), and results were more than one standard deviation below the group mean.

The important point to note was that data were collected to substantiate that this child does not have acoustic access to speech as it might occur in a typical classroom environment. The audiologist wrote the report, but the parents needed to present the report to the school principal and advocate for their child. Based on documentation of lack of acoustic access, the child received a classroom amplification system as part of a Section 504 plan. Furthermore, she was scheduled to receive an MFE to determine the need for additional services.

SUMMARY

The purpose of this chapter has been to show that there is both a philosophical and a legal framework to support the use of sound field technology in general and special education classrooms.

Philosophically, the concept of universal design supports the use of sound field technology in general education classrooms, in a preemptive fashion, to allow acoustic accessibility for diverse populations of learners.

Legally, special education legislation would allow sound field systems to be recommended for a specific child following compelling documentation of need. In addition to IDEA, the Technology-Related Assistance Act could be a source of funding for the technology.

Finally, sound field amplification seems to mesh perfectly with the NCLB of 2001. School districts are desperate to find means of improving AYP for their students. By improving the signal-to-noise ratio and enhancing acoustic accessibility, sound field technology can provide the evidence-based outcomes needed for school districts to be in compliance with NCLB.

DISCUSSION TOPICS

1. Distinguish the universal design paradigm from the special education case-by-case treatment paradigm.
2. How does the above distinction apply to sound field technology?
3. What audiologic services and treatment is a child entitled to by law?
4. How do Section 504 and IDEA differ?
5. How can the need for sound field systems be documented?
6. How can NCLB and AYP apply to the use of sound field technology in general education classrooms?

REFERENCES

Ackerhalt, A. H., & Wright, E. R. (2003). Do you know your child's special education rights? *Volta Voices, 10*(3), 4–6.

Berg, F. S. (1993). *Acoustics and sound systems in schools.* Clifton Park, NY: Thomson Delmar Learning.

Bowe, F. G. (2000). Universal design in education: Teaching nontraditional students. Westport, CT: Bergin & Garvey.

Bremer, C. D., Clapper, A. T., Hitchcock, C., Hall, T., & Kachgal, M. (2002). Universal design: A strategy to support students' access to the general education curriculum. *Information Brief, 1*(3), 1–5.

Browder, D. M., & Spooner, F. (2003). Potential benefits of the adequate yearly progress provision of NCLB for students with significant disabilities. *TASH Connections,* October, 12–17.

Fisher, L. I. (1985). Learning disabilities and auditory processing. In R. J. VanHattum (Ed.). *Administration of speech-language services in the schools* (pp. 231–292). Providence, RI: College Hill Press.

Flexer, C. (1999). *Facilitating hearing and listening in young children* (2nd ed.). Clifton Park, NY: Thomson Delmar Learning.

Keith, R. W. (2000). *SCAN-C: Test of auditory processing abilities in children* (Rev. ed.). San Antonio, TX: The Psychological Corporation.

LeRoy, B., & Kulik, N. (2003). Who's there? Students in inclusive educational settings. *TASH Connections,* October, 26–28.

No Child Left Behind Act. (2001). Education. Intergovernmental Relations. 20 USC 6301 *et. seq.* note.

President's Commission on Excellence in Special Education. (2002). *A new era: Revitalizing special education for children and their families.* Washington, DC: U.S. Department of Education.

Rehabilitation Act Amendments. (1992). P.L. 102-569. (1992, October 29). *United States Statutes at Large, 106,* 4344–4488.

Rehabilitation Act. (1973). P.L. 93-112. (1973, September 26). *United States Statutes at Large, 87,* 355–394.

Ruppmann, J. (2003). No child left behind: What it might mean for students with significant disabilities. *TASH Connections,* October, 5–7.

Seaver, L. (2003). A question of automatic eligibility: Does my deaf/HH child need an IEP? *Educational Audiology Review, 20*(3), 25–27.

Technology-Related Assistance to Individuals with Disabilities Act. (1988). P.L. 100-407, 29 U.S.C.; 2201 *et seq.* (1997).

Turnbull, H. R., Turnbull, A. P., Wehmeyer, M. L., & Park, J. (2003). A quality of life framework for special education outcomes. *Remedial and Special Education, 24*(2), 67–74.

Universal design: Ensuring access to the general education curriculum. (1999). *Research Connections in Special Education, 5,* 1–2.

U.S. Department of Education (1995). Seventeenth annual report to Congress on the implementation of the individuals with disabilities education act. Washington, DC: U.S. Government Printing Office.

U.S. Department of Health, Education, and Welfare. (1977, August 23). Rules and regulations for the administration of the education of all handicapped children act. *Federal Register* (Part IV), 42, 163.

Wehmeyer, M. L., Lance, G. D., & Bashinski, S. (2002). Promoting access to the general curriculum for students with mental retardation: A multi-level model. *Education and Training in Mental Retardation and Developmental Disabilities, 37*(3), 223–234.

INDEX